FINE-NEEDLE ASPIRATION CYTODIAGNOSIS
A COLOR ATLAS

CARLO RAVETTO

PAOLO BOCCATO

FINE-NEEDLE ASPIRATION CYTODIAGNOSIS

A COLOR ATLAS

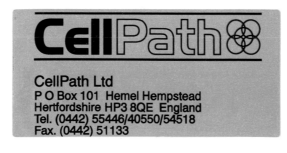

CellPath Ltd
P O Box 101 Hemel Hempstead
Hertfordshire HP3 8QE England
Tel. (0442) 55446/40550/54518
Fax. (0442) 51133

PICCIN/BUTTERWORTHS

Carlo Ravetto, M.D.
Head of Cytology Section, Busto Arsizio Hospital, Varese, Italy

Paolo Boccato, M.D., M.I.A.C.
Head of the Institute of Pathological Anatomy, San Donà di Piave Hospital, Venezia, Italy

Piccin Nuova Libraria, S.P.A., Padua, Italy.
Butterworths, London, Boston, Durban, Singapore, Sydney, Toronto, Wellington

British Library Cataloguing in Publication Data

Ravetto, Carlo
  Fine needle aspiration cytodiagnosis.
  1. Diagnosis, Cytologic   2. Biopsy, Needle
  I. Title   II. Boccato, Paolo
  III. Atlante di citodiagnostica per aspirazione con ago
  sottile.
  English
  616.07'582   RB43

  ISBN 88-299-0085-0 (PICCIN)
       0-407-01054-8 (BUTTERWORTHS)

Printed in Italy

Preface

This atlas of cytodiagnosis using fine-needle aspiration is first of all intended for clinicians and aims to present the diagnostic results, usually obtained in a few minutes, without anesthesia, from small quantities of fluid aspirated from palpable or non-palpable lesions.

The cases reported cover a wide series of diseases ranging from the most to least common ones met in clinical practice; in some cases the cytological picture is diagnostic, in others a tissue section procedure is required. In the latter case, however, fine-needle aspiration already allows classification into one of the well-defined sections of pathology (tumoral, inflammatory, malformative, degenerative etc.).

This atlas is, of course, also intended for pathologists: perhaps those already practicing this technique may find the "not-yet-met" case or appreciate some peculiar aspects in the differential diagnosis of the most difficult cases.

Colleagues, unfamiliar with this branch of anatomic pathology, will probably be struck (the authors, at least, hope so!) by the peculiarity of this diagnostic procedure where, unlike in classical cytodiagnosis, a first view at low magnification and the structural indications are often highly meaningful, in what could be defined an "almost histologic cytology".

The "text" has deliberately been limited to introduction, notes of technique and figure captions; cytological criteria for differential diagnosis have been inserted where appropriate.

The style of this atlas is that of a collection of images exhibited during a hypothetical polythematic slide seminar, accompanied by a summary of the comments on each case.

C. Ravetto and P. Boccato

Author's note: All the magnifications mentioned in the text refer to the original magnification.

CONTENTS

1

EQUIPMENT AND TECHNIQUE

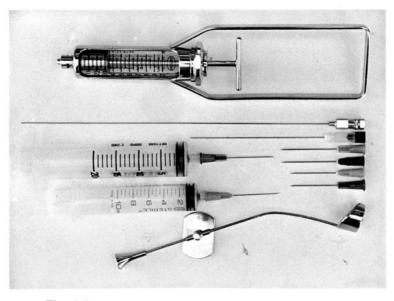

Fig. 1.1
The equipment necessary for the performance of fine-needle aspiration biopsy is limited and quite inexpensive. It consists of fine-needles usually 22-23 gauge wide, both short and long, (10 or) 20 ml syringes and an important device, the syringe holder, specially designed to allow the performance of puncture and aspiration with one hand. For transrectal and transvaginal aspiration, the Franzén guide applied to the palpating finger is a useful adjunct, which allows precise localization and aspiration from the selected site (e.g. prostatic, adnexal and parametrial masses)

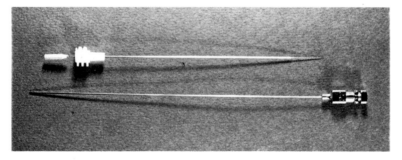

Fig. 1.2
Fine-needle aspiration biopsy of deep nodules, localized with the aid of subsidiary techniques (fluoroscopy, lymphography, angiography, echotomography, axial computerized tomography), is performed with long needles, 22-23 gauge wide and 15 or 20 cm long. With hard nodules the Nordenström needle (Rotex II) is useful because the screw-form of the end of its mandrin allows fragments of tissue to be obtained. The mandrins of the other long needles increase their rigidity and avoid possible contamination during introduction of the needle into the lesion.

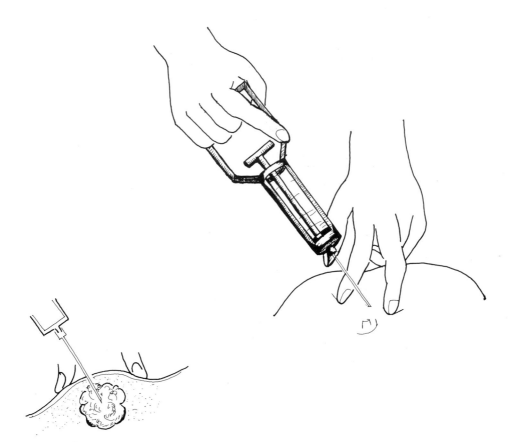

Fig. 1.3
The nodule which is to be punctured must be localized
and immobilized. It is gripped firmly between two fingers,
in the "one hand grip" technique, or delimitated between
four fingers, when the help of an assistant is available.

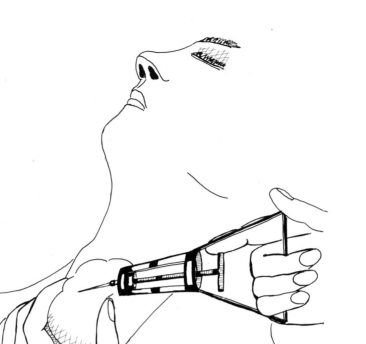

Fig. 1.4
When the nodule has been immobilized, the needle is introduced into the lesion with a rapid, precise movement; no anesthesia is required. The operator is aware of the needle's entry into the nodule when he/she encounters a more solid consistency with respect to the surrounding tissues or if the lesion is cystic. If in doubt, careful movement of the nodule causes synchronous movement of the needle, if this is correctly positioned, in the nodule.

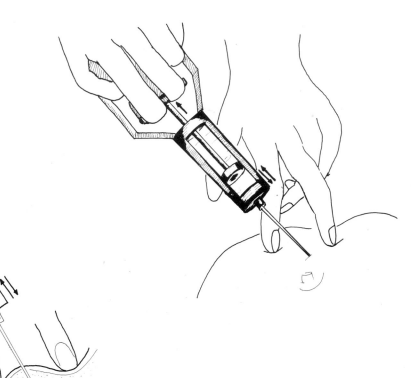

Fig. 1.5
When the needle has entered the palpable lesion, the
piston of the syringe is retracted, thus creating a vacuum.
The needle is moved back and forth, and into different
areas of the lesion. Longer aspiration is required, if the
lesion is fibrotic, shorter if it is highly vascularized. In
any case, aspiration must be stopped as soon as any
bloody material appears in the syringe.
In cystic nodules, aspiration should be continued until
no more liquid can be removed; thereafter thorough
palpation is mandatory to exclude the possibility of a
residual palpable lump; should any remaining lump be
found, a second fine-needle aspiration must be performed.

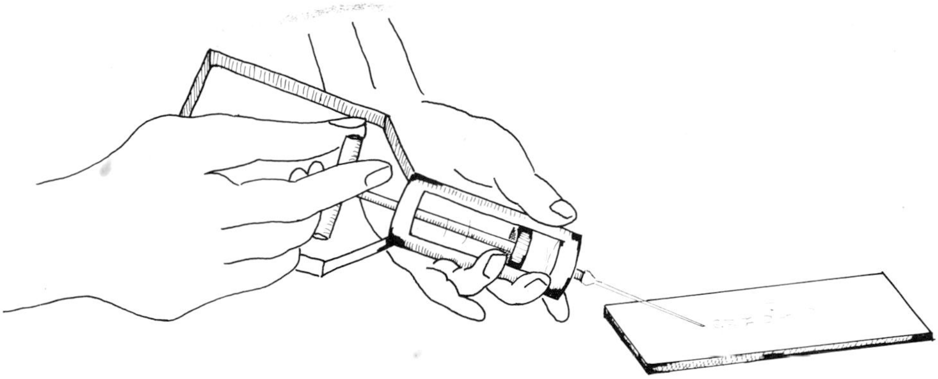

Fig. 1.6
Before the needle is withdrawn, aspiration is stopped by
releasing the piston. After withdrawal, the needle is
disconnected from the syringe, the piston retracted and
the needle reconnected. The material collected in the
needle is carefully expressed onto a glass slide. This
material usually forms a thick, variably hematic drop. If
the aspirated material is scanty, the needle is rinsed with
saline (or Hanks' fluid); this fluid is then processed by
centrifugation (or cytocentrifugation).

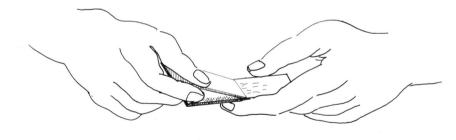

Fig. 1.7
The aspirate is smeared by flat pressure, using a second
glass-slide, but taking care to avoid excessive pressure.
The smeared material should result thicker than that of
a blood smear and similar to a bone-marrow preparation.
Fixation, by immersing the slide in 95% ethyl alcohol or
spraying the cell sample with aerosol coating fixative,
must be immediate. If the smear is air-dried, a hematologi-
cal staining technique (Wright or Pappenheim) must be
used.

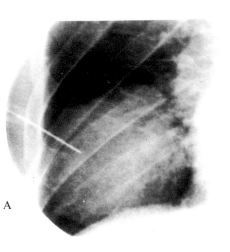

A

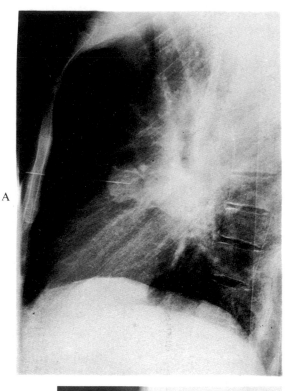

A

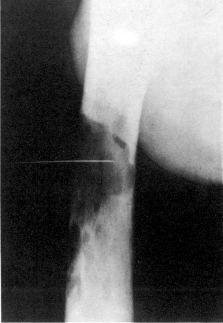

B

Fig. 1.8
Fine-needle aspiration of deep-situated, non-palpable masses can be performed under fluoroscopic guidance, namely in cases of lung (A) or skeletal system lesions (B: lytic lesion of the right femur).
Under the guidance of image-intensifier, television fluoroscopy, the exact position of the needle tip, within the lesion, can be easily assessed.

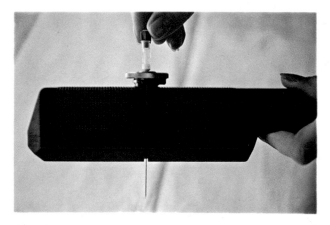

Fig. 1.9
Non-palpable chest and abdominal masses may be
visualized and localized by echography (ultrasonography).
Fine-needle aspiration of these lesions can be performed
using a special transducer with a central channel for the
needle; the transducer (connected to an ultrasonic,
real-time scanner) guides needle introduction, allows the
needle-tip's entry into the lesion to be monitored and
aspiration to be performed in a more significant area.

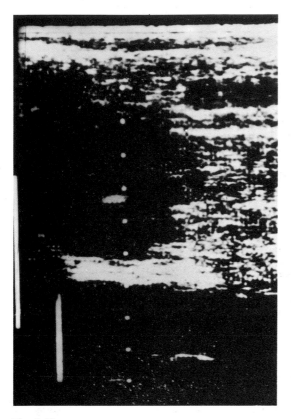

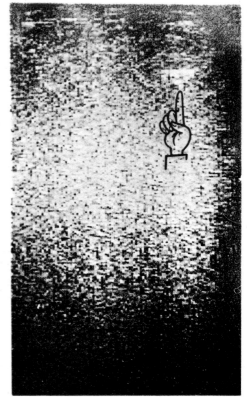

Fig. 1.10   Fig. 1.11

Figs. 1.10 and 1.11
Ultrasonic visualization of the needle-tip may be more
of less difficult. It is usually more visible in hypoechogenic
(fluid-filled) cystic structures (Fig. 1.10: partially cystic
formation in the left kidney) than in hyperechogenic
(solid) ones (Fig. 1.11: hepatic neoplasm).

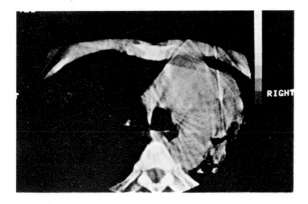

Fig. 1.12
With the use of computerized tomography (C.T.) small
nodules (less than 2 cm in diameter) can be visualized
and aspirated. In this case, monitoring is not in real time
as in ultrasonography, but is obtained by repeated scans
appropriately programmed to check the needle's path and
its correct positioning within the lesion.
In this figure, C.T. confirmation of needle position, within
a lung nodule, is shown. The whole needle is visible; the
tip is placed in the center of the lesion, which is to be
cytologically investigated.

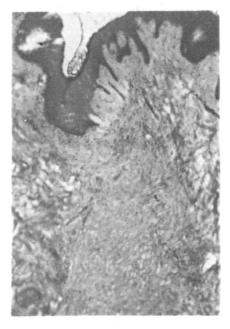

Fig. 1.13
The needling tract is usually very difficult to identify
later, histologically. Sometimes, however, if fine-needle
aspiration had been performed recently, the needling tract
may appear as a linear, hemorrhagic lesion. Less
frequently (in patients who underwent operation much
later after fine-needle aspiration), the needling tract is
represented by a linear fibrotic lesion; this picture is more
frequently observed, if (less) fine-needles of 18-19 gauge
are used, as shown in this figure.

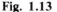

2
GENERAL FEATURES

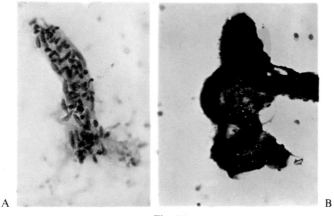

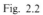

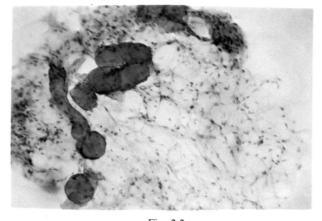

Fig. 2.2

Figs. 2.1 and 2.2
Inconclusive findings: Fig. 2.1 A: capillary; Fig. 2.1 B: sweat gland (taken with a sampling from an axillary lymphnode); Fig. 2.2: fat tissue, striped muscle fibers. (Fig. 2.1 A: Papanicolaou stain, x240; Fig. 2.1 B: M.G.G. stain, x63; Fig. 2.2: Papanicolaou stain, x63).

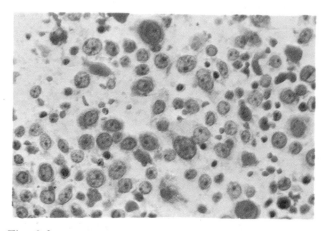

Fig. 2.3
Cellular suspension obtained by rinsing the fine-needle
with 2 ml of saline after most of the aspirate had been
expressed onto a slide. Cytologic diagnosis: *lymph node
metastasis of epidermoid carcinoma*.
(Cytocentrifuge, Papanicolaou stain, x400).

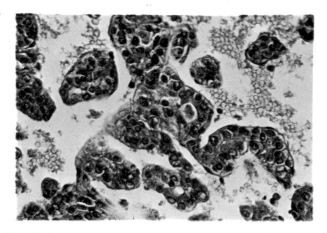

Fig. 2.4
Paraffin embedding of small fragments obtained by
fine-needle aspiration sometimes provides more precise
information about a neoplasm, since it allows an easier
diagnosis of the histological type, as in this case of
well-differentiated hepatocellular carcinoma (sample taken under ultrasonic guidance from an ultrasonically solid
nodule of the right lobe of the liver, clinically suspected
of "hepatic neoplasm").
(Papanicolaou stain, x250).

3
BRAIN

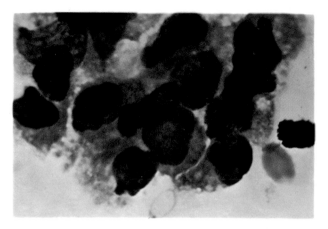

Fig. 3.1
Fine-needle aspirate from a brain neoplasia, obtained
through ventricular puncture: sheet of round epithelial
cells, with peripheral nucleus and plurivacuolated cytoplasm.
A diagnosis of ***metastasis from adenocarcinoma*** was made
(unspecified origin).
(M.G.G. stain, x1250).

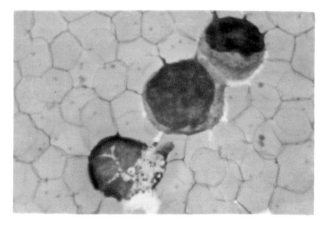

Fig. 3.2
Fine-needle aspirate from a brain "cyst" (material
obtained through the fontanelle); the two upper, round-
shaped cells (with huge nuclei, anisonucleosis and
irregular clumping of the chromatin) were judged malignant. (Tissue section diagnosis: astrocytoma).
(M.G.G. stain, x1250).

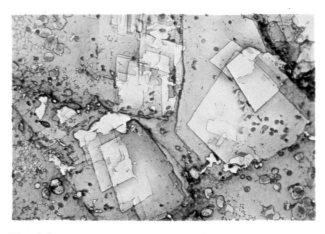

Fig. 3.3
Fine-needle aspirate from a "cystic" supersellar neoplasia
(material obtained through transnasal puncture): choleste-
rol crystals and numerous inflammatory cells. (Elsewhere
in the slide anucleated, cornified cells were present). A
cytologic diagnosis of **craniopharyngioma** was made.
(Papanicolaou stain, x250).

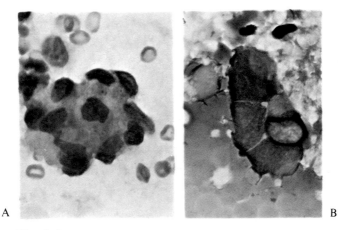

A   B

Fig. 3.4
Intraoperative, fine-needle aspirates from brain tumors
classified as **well-differentiated** (A) and **poorly-differentiated** (B) **astrocytomas**.
The nuclei, in A, are of even size; the cytoplasm with
indistinct edges is quite large with microvacuolisation.
The nuclear size in B is much greater than that of the
cells depicted in A; nuclear-cytoplasmic ratio is remarka-
bly increased. The chromatin is unevenly distributed.
(M.G.G. stain, x600).

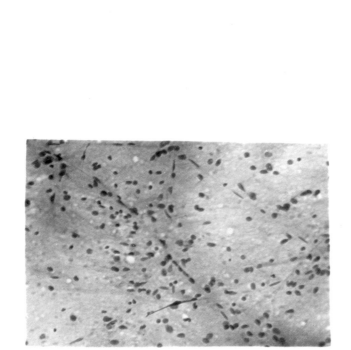

Fig. 3.5
Fine-needle aspirate, performed through a cranial burr hole, from a brain lesion, and monitored with computerized tomography: the material collected shows a rich fibrillar and relatively monomorphic cellular component. A diagnosis of **well-differentiated astrocytoma** was made (histologically confirmed).
(M.G.G. stain, x125)

4

EYE AND ORBIT

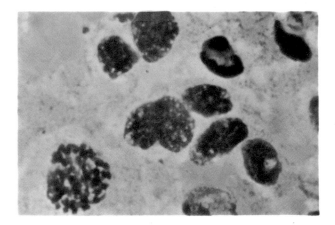

Fig. 4.1
Fine-needle aspirate from an orbital (bilateral) lesion, diagnosed as **neuroblastoma** (the primary neoplasm was in a suprarenal gland). The malignant cells are fairly monomorphic, forming an incomplete rosette. The nuclei are ovoid with some peripherically located degenerative vacuoles. See (neuroblast in) mitosis (bottom, left). (M.G.G. stain, x1250).

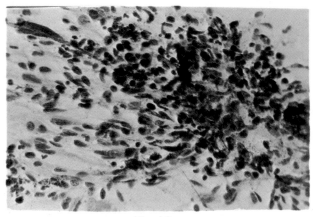

Fig. 4.2

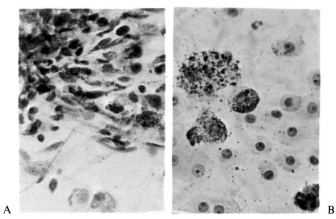

A

B

Fig. 4.3

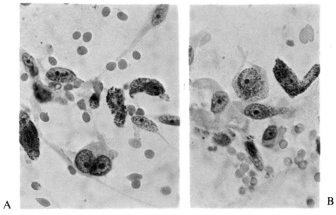

A

B

Fig. 4.4

Figs. 4.2, 4.3 and 4.4
Fine-needle aspirates (performed in the operating room
before surgery) from neoplasm of the posterior chamber
(Figs. 4.2 and 4.3) and of the ciliary body (Fig. 4.4). In
these three cases, a preoperative cytological diagnosis of
malignant melanoma was made according to an "immediate" staining procedure: wet fixed smears (in 95%
ethanol for a few seconds) were stained in Harris
hematoxylin for two minutes, rinsed in tap water and
placed under a coverslip, without mounting medium.
(The same preparations restained with Papanicolaou stain
are depicted).
In Fig. 4.2 and in Fig. 4.3 (A): *spindle-cells, malignant
melanoma;* in Fig. 4.3 (B) and in Fig. 4.4: *epithelioid,
malignant melanoma.*
(Figs. 4.2, 4.3, 4.4: Papanicolaou stain – Fig. 4.2 and Fig.
4.3 (A): x63; Fig. 4.3 (B) and Fig. 4.4: x250).

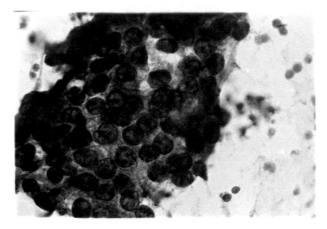

Figs. 4.5
Fine-needle aspirate from an intra-ocular choroidal mass, performed under indirect ophthalmoscopic control. The aspiration was performed through a transvitreous approach, after inserting the fine-needle in the pars plana on the side opposite the lesion. The material collected is clearly epithelial in type (cohesive round cells, with a high nuclear/cytoplasmic ratio, thickened nuclear membrane and prominent nucleoli). A diagnosis of *ocular metastasis from adenocarcinoma* was made (compatible with a breast origin). This figure demonstrates the only (apparently) metastasis originally detected (by computerized tomography) in a subject already submitted to mastectomy because of intraductal infiltrating carcinoma. (Papanicolaou stain, x630).

5

THYROID

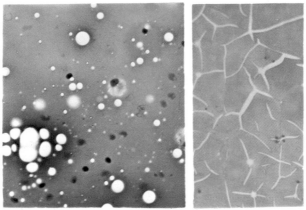

A   B

Fig. 5.1
A: This preparation was made with yellow viscid fluid aspirated from a cold thyroid node. An amorphous background consisting of colloid, with hollow areas, sparse naked nuclei of follicular cells and histiocytes can be seen. This picture is compatible with *colloidocystic goiter;* such a lesion is not neoplastic and does not necessitate surgical treatment (unless to alleviate compression on the trachea or for aesthetic reasons).
B: Sometimes characteristic splitting can be seen in the colloid.
(A: M.G.G. stain, x125; B: Papanicolaou stain, x250).

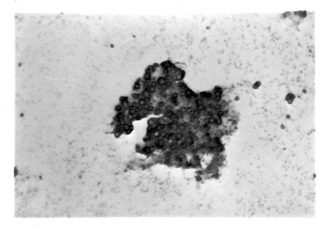

Fig. 5.2
Fine-needle aspiration from a cold thyroid node; the extracted fluid (brown-red) was cytocentrifuged; note partially lysed, red blood cells in the background, and coagulated material together with spherical calcified particles, in the midfield.
This picture may represent the cytological counterpart of a pseudocystic structure which has formed in an old hemorrhagic lesion (tissue section diagnosis: *hemorrhagic pseudocyst in nodular, colloid goiter*).
(Papanicolaou stain, x63).

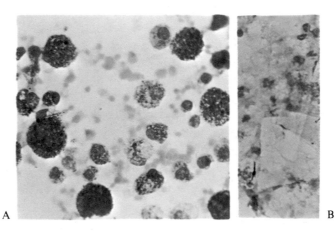

A   B

Fig. 5.3
A: Cytocentrifuge preparation of a fluid (brown) aspirated
from a cold thyroid nodule: note red blood cells and
hemosiderin-laden macrophages.
B: Cholesterin crystals and hemosiderin-laden macrophages.
This cytological picture indicates a *"pseudocystic lesion"*,
formed in an old, hemorrhagic lesion.
(A: M.G.G. stain, x250; B: M.G.G. stain, x250).

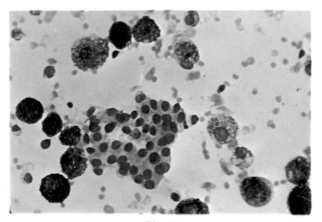

Fig. 5.4

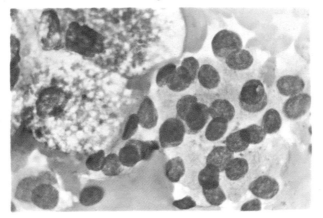

Fig. 5.5

Figs. 5.4 and 5.5
Cytocentrifuge preparations of a (brown) fluid aspirated from a cold thyroid nodule; note some hemosiderin-laden macrophages and a few follicular cells. If these are numerous, this would indicate a *cyst from an old hemorrhagic lesion, next to (or in) a follicular "neoplasm".*
(Fig. 5.4: M.G.G. stain, x250; Fig. 5.5: M.G.G. stain, x600).

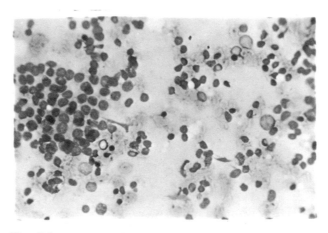

Fig. 5.6
Fine-needle aspirate from a solitary thyroid nodule;
copious mature lymphocytes (as in lymph node puncture)
and a sheet of isometric follicular cells. A diagnosis of
"lymphocytic juvenile thyroiditis" was made. On account
of the nodular aspect of the lesion, a malignant lymphoma
could only be ruled out after the cytological picture had
been confirmed with two successive aspirates. Unlike in
Hashimoto's thyroiditis, where, moreover, the gland is
symmetrical enlarged, there are no oxyphilic cells.
(M.G.G. stain, x63).

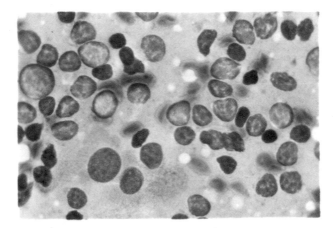

Fig. 5.7
Hashimoto's thyroiditis: note lymphocytes (which have
replaced colloid follicles), cells from germinal centres and
a few oncocytes (Hürthle cells, Askanazy cells).
(M.G.G. stain, x600).

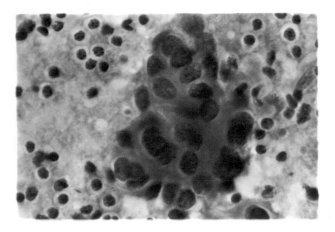

Fig. 5.8
Hashimoto's thyroiditis: cluster of swollen follicular cells
on a background of lymphoid cells. This lesion can be
differentiated from a carcinoma since the nuclear structure
is fairly regular and there are at least five times as many
lymphoid cells as epithelial cells.
(Papanicolaou stain, x400).

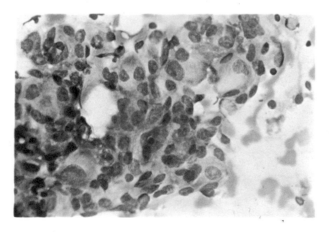

Fig. 5.9
Fine-needle aspirate from a painful asymmetrically
enlarged thyroid, in a subject affected by an influenza-like
syndrome (elevated erythrosedimentation ratio). Inflammatory cells (lymphocytes and neutrophils) together with
a cluster of swollen oncocytic-like, multilayered follicular
cells, demonstrating anisocytosis, small nucleoli and loss
of polarity.
A diagnosis of ***acute non-suppurative thyroiditis (early***
phase of de Quervain's subacute thyroiditis) was made.
Favorable outcome (after steroid therapy).
(M.G.G. stain, x250).

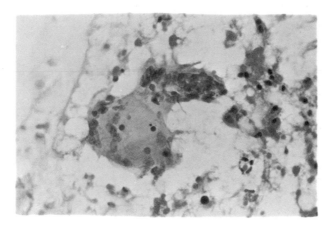

Fig. 5.10
Histiocytic, foreign body-like, giant-cell in the fine-needle
aspirate from a case of *de Quervain's thyroiditis (granulomatous pseudotubercular thyroiditis)*.
This must be differentiated from papillary carcinoma, in
which the aspirates demonstrate similar multinucleated
giant-cells (see Figs. 5.26 and 5.27), in about half of the
cases.
(Papanicolaou stain, x250).

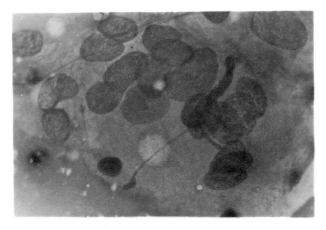

Fig. 5.11
De Quervain's granulomatous thyroiditis: at a higher
magnification than in Figure 5.10, the histiocytic charac-
ter of the multinucleated giant-cell is more obvious. Note
the round or more often ovoid, irregularly polarized
nuclei, sometimes superposed.
(M.G.G. stain, x600).

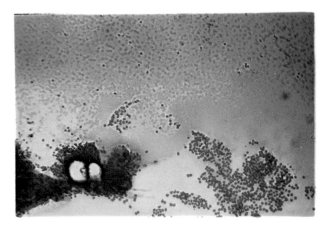

Fig. 5.12
Fine-needle aspirate from a solitary cold thyroid nodule:
note colloid in the background and many follicular cells
forming cohesive sheets. This could indicate *macro-
microfollicular "neoplasm" or nodular colloidocystic
goiter, next to a follicular neoplasm.*
(M.G.G. stain, x63).

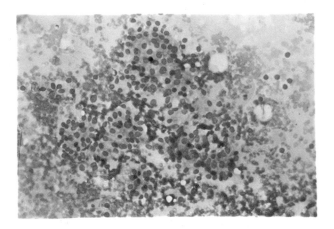

Fig. 5.13
This preparation, observed at a low magnification, was
obtained with material aspirated from a cold thyroid
nodule: note red blood cells in the background and lack
of colloid; many epithelial cells are arranged in a
microfollicular pattern. *Follicular "neoplasm"* is diagnosed and a hemithyroidectomy is indicated. Benign
follicular neoplasms are cytologically undistinguishable
from well-differentiated adenocarcinomas.
The final diagnosis must be made on the surgical
specimen, examining the largest possible number of cell
blocks, in order to identify capsular or vascular invasion.
These aspects are characteristic of malignancy (well-
differentiated adenocarcinoma).
(M.G.G. stain, x63).

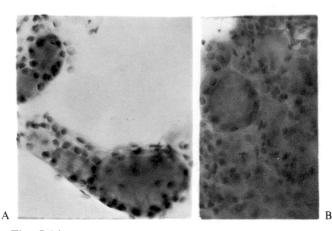

Fig. 5.14
Note in A and B, the histologic-like aspect of fragments
collected from a *follicular "neoplasm"*; the structure of
follicles containing colloid is well-preserved.
(A, B: Papanicolaou stain, x100).

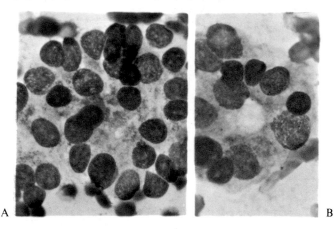

Fig. 5.15
A, B: The cytologic features are similar to those of the
previous slide. At a higher magnification, note the
microfollicular arrangement of the cells. There is slight
anisonucleosis and coarse chromatin. The cytoplasm
appears gray-blue with no distinct boundaries. In this
lesion (which could also be a well-differentiated adenocarcinoma), the cellular atypias are less marked than those
usually found in inflammatory lesions (i.e. Hashimoto's
thyroiditis, acute non-suppurative thyroiditis).
(A, B: M.G.G. stain, x600; x600).

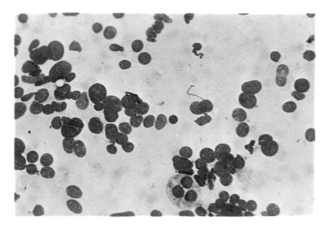

Fig. 5.16
Fine-needle aspirate from a solitary cold thyroid nodule: there is marked anisonucleosis in naked nuclei, deriving from follicular cells. There is no follicular arrangement. The tissue section diagnosis of this *follicular "neoplasm"* was *normo-microfollicular adenoma.*
Therefore, in this case, the structural and nuclear atypias were not accompanied by histological signs of malignancy. (M.G.G. stain, x250).

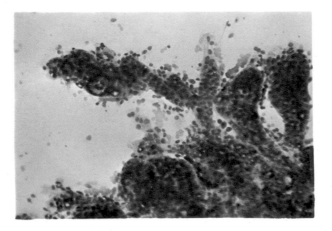

Fig. 5.17
Fine-needle aspirate from a solitary cold thyroid nodule: note no colloid and many cohesive epithelial fragments, sometimes arranged in a trabecular pattern. A diagnosis of *follicular "neoplasm" (possibly trabecular or embryonal type)* was made. In the surgical specimen (from hemithyroidectomy) aspects of plurifocal capsular invasion were noted. The patient underwent a residual hemithyroidectomy for *trabecular adenocarcinoma.*
(M.G.G. stain, x63).

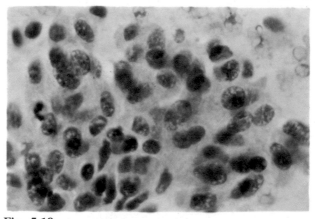

Fig. 5.18
Fine-needle aspirate from a palpable cold thyroid node.
Note a cluster of columnar epithelial cells and microfollicular arrangement. There is hypercellularity, superposition and loss of polarity. The nuclei demonstrate irregular,
thickened membranes and bounding, clumped chromatin.
In these cases, there is, cytologically, a high suggestion
of malignancy *(follicular adenocarcinoma)* even if tissue
section is required for the final diagnosis. A cytologic
diagnosis of possible malignancy must be made on the
structural aspect of the fragments and not on single
atypical cells. (In this case the diagnosis of follicular
adenocarcinoma was confirmed on tissue section).
(Papanicolaou stain, x600).

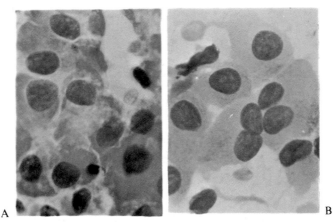

A   B

Fig. 5.19
A: Fine-needle aspirate from a *Hürthle cell tumor* (so
called *oncocytoma*). The cells are large and cohesive; the
cytoplasm is abundant and contains eosinophilic, fairly
evident granules (in Papanicolaou preparation); the
nucleus is usually ovoid, with a delicate or coarse
chromatin. An eosinophilic (or cyanophilic), sometimes
prominent nucleolus is occasionally present.
B: In M.G.G. preparations, the cells, which are larger
than those observed in Papanicolaou slides, show less
evident cytoplasmic granules.
(A: Papanicolaou stain, x600; B: M.G.G. stain, x600).

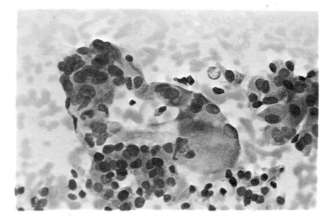

Fig. 5.20
Fine-needle aspirate from a *fairly dedifferentiated oncocy-tic neoplasm:* note anisochariosis and anisonucleosis in Hürthle cells, in some parts arranged in a microfollicular pattern. The multinucleated cells are probably polyploid oncocytes. According to Lopes Cordozo these neoplasms should always be considered malignant.
(M.G.G. stain, x100).

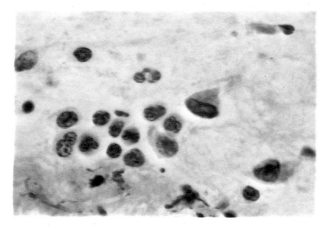

Fig. 5.21
Fine-needle aspirate from thyroid lump, classified as an *anaplastic, small-cell carcinoma*. Note some small lym-phocytic-like cells; the cytoplasm is scanty, the nuclear membrane thickened and the chromatin coarse. These cells are intermingled with larger ones, some of which are multinucleated, with prominent nucleoli and abun-dant cytoplasm.
(Papanicolaou stain, x600).

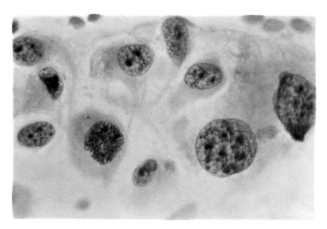

Fig. 5.22
Fine-needle aspirate from an **anaplastic, giant-cell carcinoma** of the thyroid. The malignant cells are larger than
those in Figure 5.21, and appear isolated, pleomorphic,
ovoid or round; the nuclear membranes are thickened
with coarsely clumped chromatin and prominent nucleoli.
(Papanicolaou stain, x600).

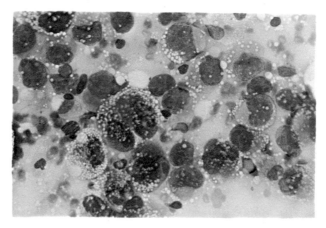

Fig. 5.23
Fine-needle aspirate from a thyroid node; the cytological
picture clearly indicates malignancy (epithelial); note very
marked anisonucleosis, bizarre and multiple nuclei, many
prominent eosinophilic nucleoli. One cell is five times
larger than the other tumor cells.
A diagnosis of **undifferentiated, giant-cell type carcinoma
(thyroid?)** was made; similar cells were also observed in
sputum specimens. Chest x-ray films demonstrated a
nodular lesion, compatible with malignant neoplasm.
In this case, the origin of the neoplasia (? thyroid; ? lung)
could not be stated. From a cytological point of view an
anaplastic, giant-cell carcinoma of the thyroid may be
undistinguishable from that of the lung.
(M.G.G. stain, x400).

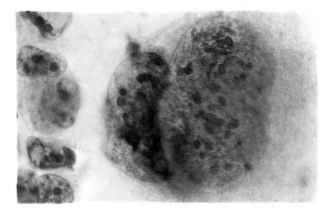

Fig. 5.24
The same case as in Figure 5.23, in a Papanicolaou
preparation. Very marked anisocytosis, bizarre nuclei,
irregular chromatin network, prominent nucleoli.
(x630).

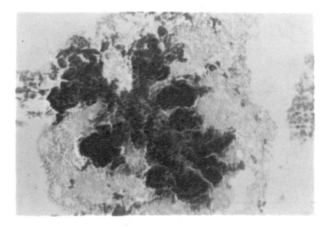

Fig. 5.25
Fine-needle aspirate from cold thyroid nodule; the
neoplastic, multilayered cells constitute a structure with
fronds and papillary groups, with a fairly evident collagen
core. There is a very marked overlapping of the nuclei
at the periphery of the fronds. A cytological diagnosis of
papillary adenocarcinoma of the thyroid was made.
(Tissue sections revealed papillary carcinoma).
(Papanicolaou stain, x100).

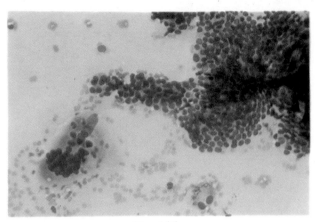

Fig. 5.26

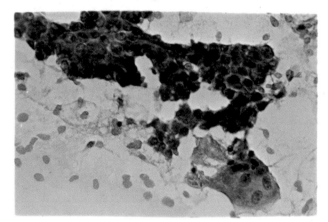

Fig. 5.27

Figs. 5.26 and 5.27
Fine-needle aspirate from a thyroid nodule, observed at
low magnification: note papillary structure (in Fig. 5.26
a fibrous – vascular axis is evident; a giant multinucleated
histiocyte (bottom, left) represents a frequent aspect of
thyroid *papillary adenocarcinomas:* this diagnosis was
histologically confirmed).
(Fig. 5.26: M.G.G. stain, x125; Fig. 5.27: Papanicolaou
stain, x125).

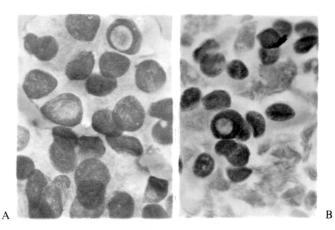

A   B

Fig. 5.28
A, B: Fine-needle aspirate from a cold thyroid nodule.
The epithelial cells derived from the papillary covering
appear isolated or irregularly crowded. Two nuclei (A,
top; B, center) demonstrate a pale, round, hollow area,
circumscribed by a ring of clumped chromatin (pseudoinclusion, pseudonucleolus), due to an intranuclear
cytoplasmic invagination. This pseudoinclusion is characteristic of papillary adenocarcinoma of the thyroid, but
may also be observed, even if rarely, in medullary
carcinomas. This feature is particularly useful in the
correct diagnosis of papillary carcinomas with a follicular
pattern.
In this case, a diagnosis of ***papillary carcinoma*** of the
thyroid was made (histologically confirmed).
(A: M.G.G. stain, x600; B: Papanicolaou stain, x600).

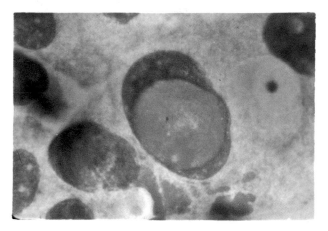

Fig. 5.29
Case similar to the previous one: pseudoinclusion
(pseudonucleolus). At a higher magnification, the periphe-
ric clumping of chromatin (karyotheca) can be seen.
(M.G.G. stain, x1250).

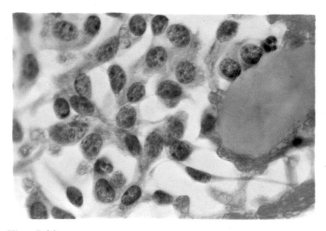

Fig. 5.30
Fine-needle aspirate from a thyroid neoplasm, cytologically classified as ***medullary carcinoma*** (histologically confirmed). The tumor cells are numerous, dispersed, spindle-type; the nuclei are round or ovoid and hyperchromatic. Note the "ialine" material identified as amyloid, on the right.
(Papanicolaou stain, x600).

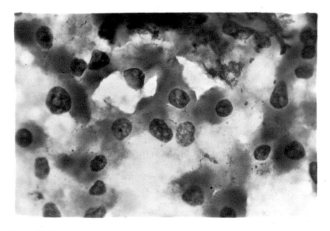

Fig. 5.31
Fine-needle aspirate from a thyroid neoplasm, cytologically classified as ***medullary carcinoma*** (histologically confirmed). The neoplastic cells are numerous; anisonucleosis, coarsely clumped chromatin and sometimes prominent nucleoli can be seen. The cytoplasm is gray; the Congo-red stain causes a birefringence when polarized.
(M.G.G. stain, x600).

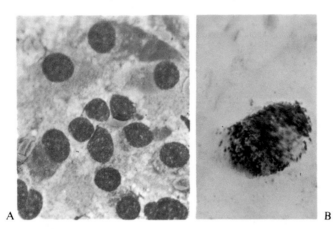

Fig. 5.32
A: Fine-needle aspirate from a thyroid neoplasm, cytologically classified as *medullary carcinoma* (histologically confirmed); in this case, the cytoplasm of the neoplastic cells demonstrates prominent red granules.
B: Medullary carcinoma of the thyroid; note neurosecretory granules in the cytoplasm of a neoplastic cell.
(A: M.G.G. stain, x600; B: Grimelius, x1250).
Note, in Figs. 5.30, 5.31 and 5.32, the marked cytological polymorphism of the medullary carcinoma of the thyroid.

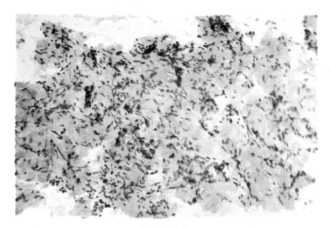

Fig. 5.33

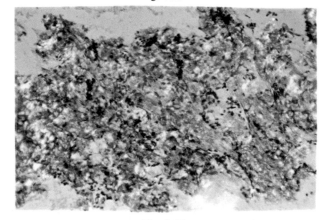

Fig. 5.34

Figs. 5.33 and 5.34
Fine-needle aspirate from an asymmetrically enlarged
thyroid, in a 25-year-old subject, with cystic fibrosis
(viscidosis). Irregular fragments of amorphous material
(green-staining with Papanicolaou method) were collected; artifactually stretched and distorted nuclei (from
follicular epithelial cells) are interspersed in this material.
Figure 5.33 shows the microscopic appearance of a slide
restained with Congo red; in Figure 5.34, note the
diagnostic "apple green" dichroic birefringence due to
diffuse ***amyloid deposits.***
(Secondary) amyloidosis is a common complication
during the course of chronic infectious processes; so
amyloidosis may occur during the course of cystic fibrosis,
especially in those patients who survive for a long time.
(Figs. 5.33 and 5.34: Congo red, x250; Fig. 5.34, in
polarized light).

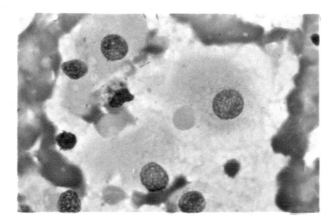

Fig. 5.35
Fine-needle aspirate from a cold thyroid nodule: the cells are round or ovoid, non-cohesive; the nuclear-cytoplasmic ratio is favourable; the cytoplasm is large, clear.
Such a picture is compatible both with a *primary, clear-cell carcinoma of the thyroid* and with a *metastatic malignancy from a clear-cell adenocarcinoma of the kidney*. In routine cytological preparations, the two neoplasms are undistinguishable; the renal origin may only be established on the basis of cytoplasmic positivity to the periodic acid-Schiff stain (not resistant to diastase). (M.G.G. stain, x600).

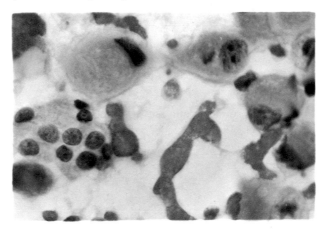

Fig. 5.36
In this fine-needle aspirate of a thyroid nodule one can observe large, dyshesive tumor cells together with a sheet of regular follicular cells. This picture, where normal structures of the thyroid are still present, would suggest a metastatic rather than a primary tumor.
In this case a diagnosis of *metastatic breast carcinoma to the thyroid* was made, on the basis of the clinical data. (Papanicolaou stain, x600).

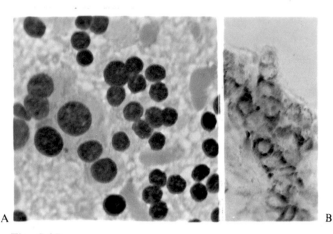

Fig. 5.37
Fine-needle aspirate (performed under ultrasonic guidance) from a non-palpable nodule of the thyroid gland region (diameter less than 1 cm). The cytological picture in A is compatible with a thyroid follicular "neoplasm" characterized by some anisonucleosis. The clinical and laboratory picture, however, suggested a parathyroid tumor. The material collected (in B) shows argyrophilic cytoplasmic granules. A diagnosis of *parathyroid adenoma* was made (histologically confirmed).
(A: M.G.G., x600; B: Grimelius, x600).

6
SALIVARY GLANDS

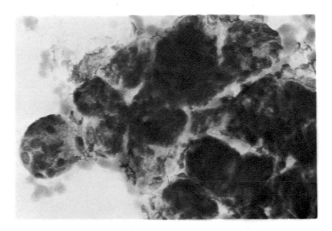

Fig. 6.1
Fine-needle aspirate from parotid: *normal serous cells*
with little, round nuclei and abundant, finely-granulated
cytoplasm. These cells constitute acini which are adherent
to an intralobular duct (not in focus) ("almost histologic
picture").
In well-differentiated acinic cell carcinomas, the morphology of the malignant cells may be cytologically undistinguishable from that of normal acinar cells, but in these
cases (see Fig. 5.12), a normal ductal-acinar structure is
never observable in fine-needle preparations.
(M.G.G. stain, x250).

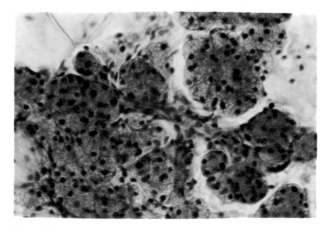

Fig. 6.2
Cytological picture superposable on Figure 6.1. In this
case, the intralobular duct, and the many acini adhering
to it are clearly evident.
(Papanicolaou stain, x250).

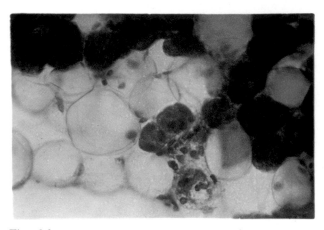

Fig. 6.3
Fine-needle aspirate from a salivary gland, characterised
by a rich fatty component in which residual isolated acini
are present. In this case, swelling of the gland really
represents an atrophic lesion (mostly due to ductal
obstruction by calculi) where large glandular areas are
replaced by fatty tissue *(sialosis).*
(Papanicolaou stain, x250).

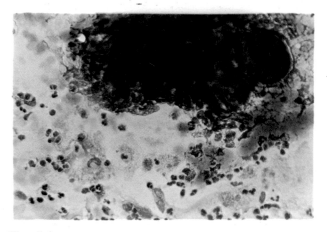

Fig. 6.4
Fine-needle aspirate from a stone-hard, painful, swollen
parotid: note numerous inflammatory cells (neutrophils,
lymphocytes and histiocytes) intermingled with acini; a
diagnosis of *subacute sialadenitis* was made. Favorable
outcome (the patient was treated with antibiotics and a
calculus was removed from the Stenone duct).
(M.G.G. stain, x250).

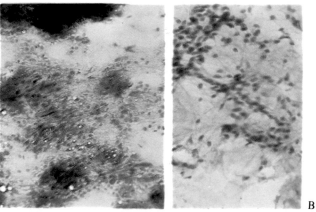

Fig. 6.5
A: Fine-needle aspirate from a swollen submandibular
gland: note extracellular mucus in mixoid, red-stained
areas and epithelial, isolated or cohesive cells. The
morphologic aspects of these cells are depicted in Figure
6.6.
B: The same case as in A. Note fibrils in a mixoid,
green-gray area, stromal and epithelial cells.
This picture corresponds to a *pleomorphic adenoma (so
called mixed tumor)* which is the commonest tumor of
the salivary grands.
(A: M.G.G. stain, x30; B: Papanicolaou stain, x125).

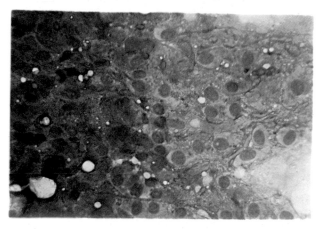

Fig. 6.6
Fine-needle aspirate from the same case as in Figure 6.5,
at a higher magnification. The neoplastic epithelial cells
show ovoid, sometimes eccentrically situated nuclei,
surrounded by gray-blue fairly abundant cytoplasm. The
mixoid, intercellular substance is characteristically fibrillar.
(M.G.G. stain, x250).

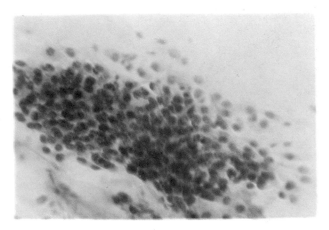

Fig. 6.7
Fine-needle aspirate from a parotid neoplasm. Monomorphic, crowded, ovoid cells constitute a solid cluster. Those more peripherically situated are isolated, with ovoid nuclei, surrounded by little pale-green cytoplasm. Elsewhere in the slide, stromal fragments were present; they did not demonstrate the fibrillar aspect of the stromal structures seen in pleomorphic adenoma.
A diagnosis of *basal cell adenoma* was made.
(Papanicolaou stain, x125).

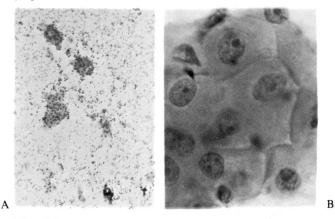

A   B

Fig. 6.8
Fine-needle aspirate from a swollen submandibulary gland, which resembled a lymph node, on clinical examination.
A: Innumerable lymphocytes and sheets of epithelial eosinophilic cells.
B: Epithelial sheet at a higher magnification. The cells are cohesive, polyhedral-shaped, with very sharp edges, ovoid nuclei, prominent nucleoli, granular cytoplasm and a favourable nuclear-cytoplasmic ratio. These cells were classified as oncocytes; a diagnosis of *Warthin's tumor (cystadenoma lymphomatosum)* was made (histologically confirmed).
(A: Papanicolaou stain, x63; B: Papanicolaou stain, x400).

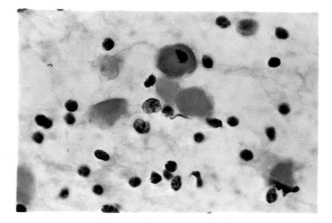

Fig. 6.9
The same case as in Figure 6.8. Innumerable lymphocytes intermingled with isolated epithelial cells, with eosinophilic or orangeophilic cytoplasm. They appear round or irregular-shaped, sometimes anucleated; sometimes a little, triangular, structureless nucleus can be seen. These cells are necrotic oncocytes aspirated from the "cemetery pools", which have formed because of regressive changes. These features may be misdiagnosed cytologically as a lymph metastasis from epidermoid carcinoma, when the aspirated lesion is erroneously believed to be a lymph node.
(Papanicolaou stain, x250).

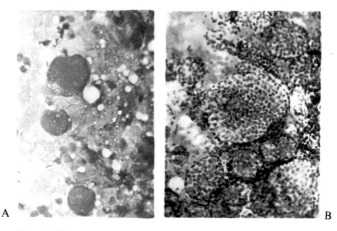

A   B

Fig. 6.10
A: Fine-needle aspirate from a parotid lump. Numerous acini embedded in a homogeneous, structureless deep red-stained substance, can be observed. Amorphous red-stained globs corresponding to "cylinders", are also present. A diagnosis of *well-differentiated adenoid cystic carcinoma (so called cylindroma)* was made (histologically confirmed).
B: The same case as in A. The round or ovoid structures correspond to globs (cylinders); they appear transparent, colorless and surrounded by carcinomatous cells.
(A: M.G.G. stain, x63; B: Papanicolaou stain, x63).

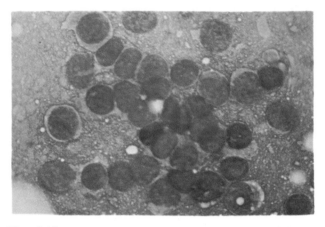

Fig. 6.11
Fine-needle aspirate from an *adenoid cystic carcinoma,
prevalently solid in type*. The cells are fairly crowded and
monomorphic; the nuclear-cytoplasmic ratio is higher
than in pleomorphic adenoma cells. The ialine material
does not form globs and is interspersed among the
neoplastic cells. In this case, the cytologic diagnosis is
more difficult than in the previous case; moreover, the
prevalently solid forms have a poorer prognosis than the
"cribriform", well-differentiated types.
(M.G.G. stain, x600).

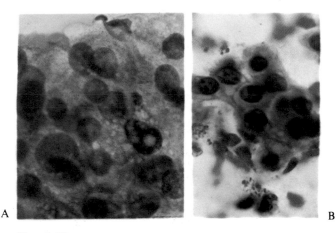

A   B

Fig. 6.12
A: Fine-needle aspirate from a parotid lump; note a fairly
monomorphic population of acinic cells, with irregular
arrangement and frequent overlapping; they do not form
acini. The nuclei are round, of different sizes, mostly
central; the cytoplasm is granular. A diagnosis of *acinic
cell carcinoma* was made (histologically confirmed).
In well-differentiated, acinic cell carcinomas, the neoplastic cells resemble normal serous cells, and, therefore, a
differentiation from a non-neoplastic lump of the salivary
gland may be very difficult. A non-neoplastic lesion is
suggested by the presence of well-formed acinic structures,
basal nuclei and ductal epithelium (it should be remembered that in well-differentiated, acinic cell carcinoma, the
lobular structure is cancelled because of the lack of ducts;
thus, in malignant lesions, a slight cytological atypia is
accompanied by a very marked structural disorder).
B: *Acinic cell carcinoma.* When compared with A, the
nuclear details are more evident. The cytoplasm is
granular. There is no tendency to form acinic structures.
(A: M.G.G. stain, x600; B: Papanicolaou stain, x600).

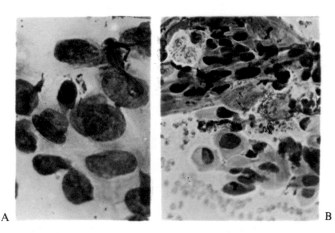

A   B

Fig. 6.13
Fine-needle aspirate from a parotid neoplasm, classified
as *moderately differentiated mucoepidermoid tumor*.
A: Epidermoid, fairly monomorphic component (larger
cells, with blue, non-foamy cytoplasm); the smaller cells,
with barely perceptible cytoplasm, are probably interme-
diate cells.
B: Cluster of tumor cells, mostly epidermoidal; a few cells
show transparent cytoplasm and eccentrically situated
nuclei (mucus secreting cells).
(A: M.G.G. stain, x600; B: Papanicolaou stain, x250).

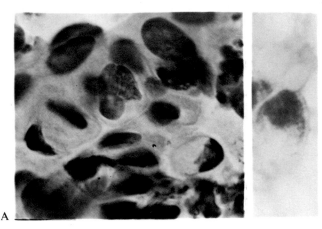

A   B

Fig. 6.14
The same case as in Figure 6.13.
A: At a higher magnification, one can observe some
mucus-secreting cells, with transparent cytoplasm and
eccentrically situated nuclei.
B: Detail of a mucus-secreting cell.
(A: Papanicolaou stain, x600; B: Mucicarmine stain,
x1250).

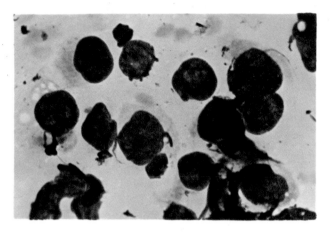

Fig. 6.15
Fine-needle aspirate from a parotid lump: dyshesive, malignant, large cells; note anisonucleosis and bizarre nuclei; the nuclear-cytoplasmic ratios are greatly increased. A diagnosis of *highly dedifferentiated, salivary gland carcinoma* was made (histologically confirmed). (M.G.G. stain, x600).

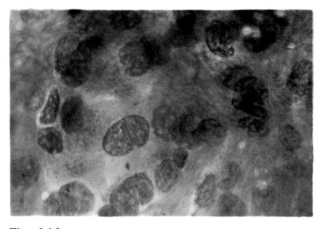

Fig. 6.16
Fine-needle aspirate from a parotid lump. Fibrillar mucus and numerous malignant cells. There is evident anisonucleosis; the nuclei are irregular in shape, cleaved and often partially overlapping. This picture suggests *malignant mixed tumor ex-pleomorphic adenoma*.
In these cases, one should perform multiple aspirates from different areas in order to correctly identify the (malignant) part of the neoplasm to be resected. (M.G.G. stain, x600).

7
LYMPH NODES

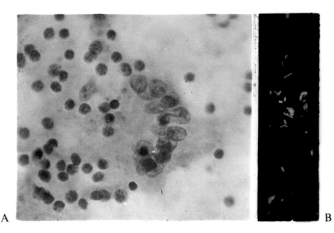

Fig. 7.1
A: Fine-needle aspirate from a cervical lymph node: note a multinucleated giant Langhans' cell, many lymphocytes and some epithelioid cells.
B: In the same lymph node aspirate, acid-fast organisms (auramin stained, observed in fluorescent light), identified as *Mycobacterium tuberculosis*, are present.
In this case, the cytological technique of fine-needle aspiration combined with a direct smear stained for acid-fast organisms, allowed an etiologic diagnosis of lymphadenopathy to be made *(tuberculous lymphadenitis)*.
(A: Papanicolaou stain, x630; B: x1250).

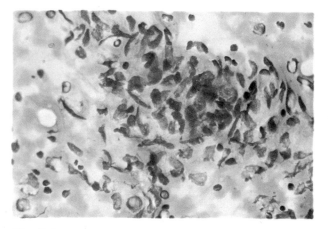

Fig. 7.2
Same case as in the previous slide. Note concentrically arranged, crowded epithelioid cells. The nuclei of the younger cells are ovoid whereas those of the oldest cells are spindle-shaped. Such a picture suggests tuberculosis, sarcoidosis or cat-scratch disease.
(M.G.G. stain, x100).

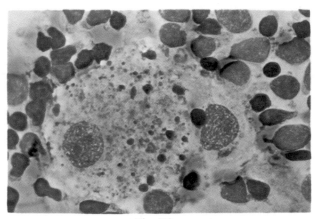

Fig. 7.3

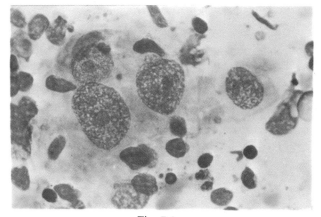

Fig. 7.4

Figs. 7.3 and 7.4
Aspirate from a nucal lymphadenopathy. Note the
variable-sized red, pink and gray-green corpuscles engul-
fed in the cytoplasm of the macrophage; some of them
are dust-like, others round, ovoid or crescent-shaped (Fig.
7.3). Some authors believe that these structures correspond, at least in part, to degenerative aspects of the
Toxoplasma gondii.
In Figure 7.4, four epithelioid cells are depicted.
This cytological picture has been considered the counterpart of a ***Piringer-Kuchinka's lymphadenitis***. The tests
for toxoplasmosis revealed high levels of serum antibo-
dies. Favorable outcome (following sulphamidic treatment, the cervical and nucal lymphadenopathies disap-
peared).
(Figs. 7.3 and 7.4: M.G.G., x630)

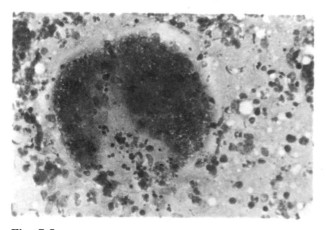

Fig. 7.5
Fine-needle aspirate from an inguinal lymph node: giant
Langhans'-like cell (note multiple peripheral nuclei) on
a background of innumerable neutrophils (the patient had
been scratched by a cat, on the homolateral leg). A
cytological diagnosis of *benign lymphoreticulosis* was
made.
(M.G.G. stain, x100).

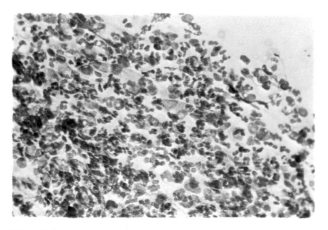

Fig. 7.6
Fine-needle aspirate from an inguinal suppurative lymphadenopathy: innumerable neutrophils intermingled
with a few epithelioid cells. A diagnosis of *suppurative
lymphadenitis* was made (this lesion was considered a
consequence of a varicose ulcer of the homolateral leg).
(M.G.G. stain, x100).

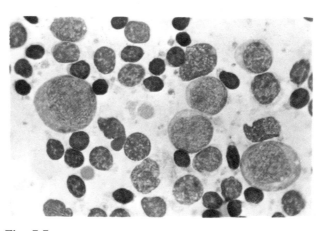

Fig. 7.7
Fine-needle aspirate from a cervical lymph node. The picture is polymorphous; note large cells with fairly basophilic cytoplasm and large, round nuclei with nucleoli (stem cells): in these cases, the cytological picture is compatible with a diagnosis of *immunologically transformed lymph node (lymph node hyperplasia)*; such an appearance may be due to quite different antigenic stimulations (bacteria, fungi, parasites, viruses, drugs).
In doubtful cases, a second fine-needle aspiration should be performed within one month, if the lymphadenopathy does not spontaneously disappear.
In the case presented, the outcome was favourable.
(M.G.G. stain, x630).

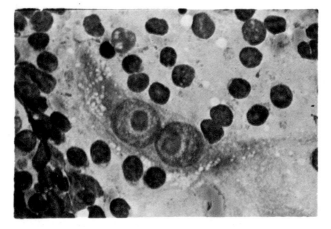

Fig. 7.8
Fine-needle aspirate from a cervical lymphadenopathy, corresponding to *lymphadenitis n.o.s. (simple lymphadenitis)*. Note one multinucleated histiocytic cell, with macronucleoli, in a background of lymphoid cells.
Favourable outcome (spontaneous disappearance of the lymphadenopathy).
(M.G.G. stain, x630).

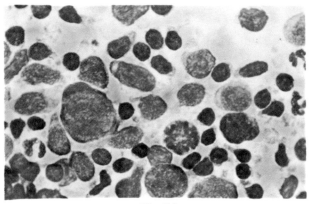

Fig. 7.9

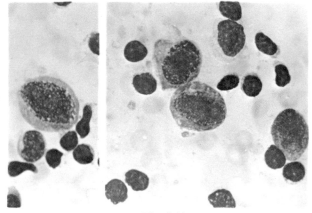

Fig. 7.10

Figs. 7.9 and 7.10
Fine-needle aspirate from a cervical lymphadenopathy; the picture is highly polymorphous. In Figure 7.9 lymphocytes intermingled with some large cells with a highly basophilic cytoplasm and peripheral pseudopodial-like elongations can be seen; note mitotic activity. In Figure 7.10, highly basophilic ovoid cells with ovoid nuclei and prominent nucleoli are depicted.

This polymorphous picture, showing mitosis in some cells, could indicate *"early" infectious mononucleosis*, which was diagnosed cytologically, in this case. After a few days, the neutrophilia in the blood smears had changed into the peculiar polymorphous features of infectious mononucleosis. The Paul-Bunnel-Davidsohn reaction (negative at the time of fine-needle aspiration) gave positive results later.
(Figs 7.9 and 7.10: M.G.G. stain, x630).

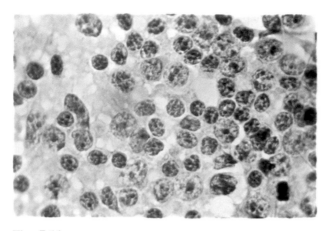

Fig. 7.11
Fine-needle aspirate from a lymph node: note monomorphic picture of cleaved cells with small nucleoli and barely
perceptible cytoplasm (centrocytes).
Lymphomatous centrocytes and those aspirated from
germinal centers are undistinguishable, and, therefore, a
cytologic diagnosis of a possible lymphoma must be based
on the almost exclusive presence of centrocytes in
preparations obtained from a satisfactory sampling.
Cytologic features similar to those seen in this slide should
lead directly to formal biopsy.
(Papanicolaou stain, x600).

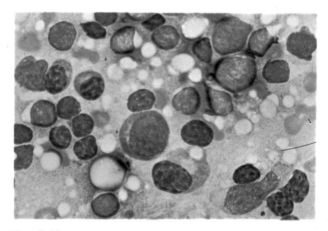

Fig. 7.12
Polymorphous picture characterized by the presence of
lymphocytes, mature plasma cells and large immature
plasmocytic cells. This feature suggests the need for an
open biopsy, since a ***lymphoplasmacytoid lymphoma is
suspected.*** (Tissue section diagnosis: lymphoplasmacytoid
lymphoma).
(M.G.G. stain, x600).

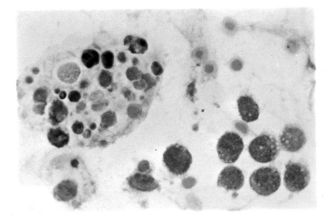

Fig. 7.13
Fine-needle aspirate from a large cervico-mandibular
lymphadenopathy: note two histiocytic cells and nine
dyshesive, monomorphic, "lymphoid" cells. The larger
histiocyte has phagocytized nuclear debris; the "lymphoid" cells show round nuclei, a thin peripheral rim of
cytoplasm, and small nuclear and cytoplasmic vacuoles.
The cytological diagnosis of a *possible Burkitt's lympho-*
ma was confirmed histologically.
(Papanicolaou stain, x600).

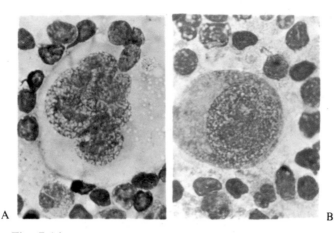

A   B

Fig. 7.14
Fine-needle aspirate from a cervical lymph node.
A: Note giant, multinucleated cell, with slight overlapping
of the nuclei, which are ovoid with eosinophilic macronucleoli. The cytoplasm is large, agranular, slightly basophilic. This cell, classified as a lacunar Reed-Sternberg cell,
is surrounded by numerous lymphocytes; one eosinophil
(bottom, left).
B: Some large (possibly Hodgkin's) cells are intermingled
with Reed-Sternberg cells, and show one round nucleus
with a nucleolus.
Lacunar Reed-Sternberg cells are usually observed together with a rich population of eosinophils; this feature is
highly suggestive of the **sclerosing nodular type of
Hodgkin's lymphoma**. (In this case the cytologic diagnosis
was histologically confirmed).
(M.G.G. stain, x630).

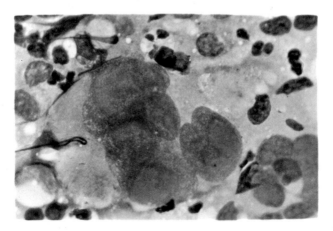

Fig. 7.15
Highly polyploid Reed-Sternberg cell in an aspirate from
Hodgkin's lymphoma, mixed cellularity type.
(M.G.G. stain, x600).

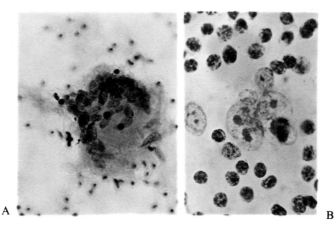

Fig. 7.16
Fine-needle aspirate from a cervical lymphadenopathy: many multinucleated Langhans'-type cells were observed (see A).
An erroneous cytologic diagnosis of granulomatous lymphadenitis (possibly tuberculous adenitis) was made. The tissue-section diagnosis was: ***Hodgkin's lymphoma with tubercle-like histiocytic reaction***. Re-examination of the cytological preparations allowed identification of very sparse Reed-Sternberg cells (see B), overlooked at the first examination.
(A, B: Papanicolaou stain, x400).

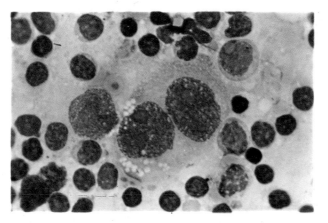

Fig. 7.17
Fine-needle aspirate from a lymph node; elsewhere in the slide, the picture allowed diagnosis of ***lymph node metastasis from epidermoid carcinoma***. In this slide, some poorly-differentiated, epidermoid cells show two nuclei with multiple macronucleoli (Sternberg-like aspect).
(M.G.G. stain, x600).

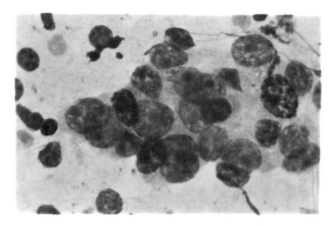

Fig. 7.18
It may sometimes be difficult to differentiate between a
lymph node metastasis from a poorly-differentiated,
epidermoid carcinoma and that from an adenocarcinoma,
because, as in this case, a large number of cohesive cells
with macronucleoli are present. In such cases, a careful
search for keratinized cells is necessary.
(M.G.G. stain, x600).

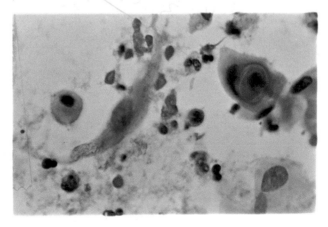

Fig. 7.19
Lymph node metastasis of a well-differentiated, epider-
moid carcinoma, with marked atypias; the cell shapes
vary from round to flattened, the cytoplasm is sometimes
cyanophilic, and sometimes amphophilic. Note the
so-called "cannibalism" (which is really an overlapping
of cells). The background is necrotic.
(Papanicolaou stain, x600).

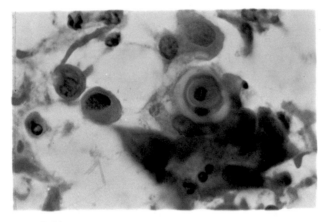

Fig. 7.20
The same case as in the previous slide; the orangiophilia
in many malignant cells is irregular; note a squamous
pearl.
(Papanicolaou stain, x600).

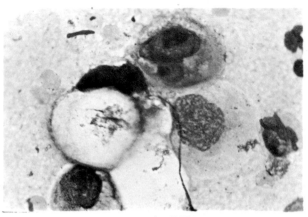

Fig. 7.21

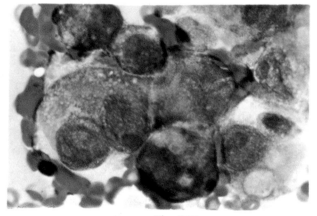

Fig. 7.22

Figs. 7.21 and 7.22
Lymph node metastasis from a mucus-secreting adenocar-cinoma; the cells are highly atypical, dyshesive, sometimes multinucleated with macronucleoli. Note, signet-ring cell in Figure 7.21 and the cell with multiple secretory vacuoles, in Figure 7.22 (bottom, right).
(Fig. 7.21: M.G.G. stain, x600; Fig. 7.22: M.G.G. stain, x600).

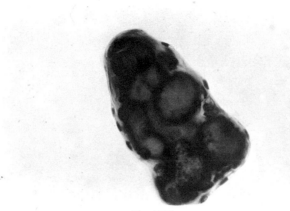

Fig. 7.23

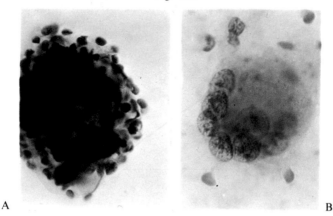

A   B

Fig. 7.24

Figs. 7.23 and 7.24
Fine-needle aspirate from a cervical "cyst" (present for
25 years). The fluid withdrawn (approximately 25 ml)
was filtered through Millipore⊙ and the collected cells
transferred onto a frozen slide, according to a modified
filter imprint technique; note in Figure 7.23 and in A of
Figure 7.24, two papillary structures, covered by monolayered epithelium; there are numerous, round, concentrically arranged, crowded structures (psammoma bodies),
in the connective axis. In B of Figure 7.24, a multinucleated giant histiocyte. A diagnosis of *lymph node metastasis
from papillary thyroid carcinoma* was made (histologically
confirmed).
(Fig. 7.23: Papanicolaou stain, x630; Fig. 7.24 A, B:
Papanicolaou stain, x630).

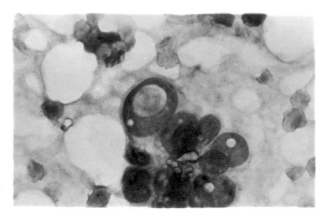

Fig. 7.25
Fine-needle aspirate from a cervical lymphadenopathy in
a patient whose thyroid gland appeared clinically normal.
Note a malignant papillary structure where the largest
cell shows a characteristic nuclear pseudoinclusion. This
feature suggests *lymph node metastasis from thyroid
papillary adenocarcinoma.* In this case, a total thyroidec-
tomy was performed and a papillary adenocarcinoma of
0.5 cm in diameter was identified.
(M.G.G. stain, x630).

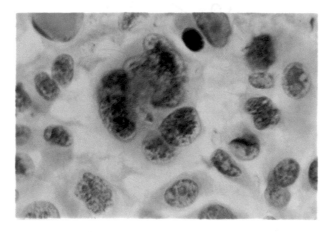

Fig. 7.26
Fine-needle aspirate from an axillary lymphadenopathy
in a patient with nodular malignant melanoma of the
homolateral forearm. *The cytological picture is clearly
one of malignancy;* the neoplastic cells are dyshesive,
round, ovoid or spindle-shaped; the nuclei irregular, often
cleaved, with thickened membrane and sometimes fairly
prominent nucleoli; in the mid-field, a giant multinucleated cell. No intra- or extracellular melanin.
If the cytologist is not aware of the clinical history
(presence of a primary melanotic malignancy), the
cytological diagnosis of *lymph node metastasis of a
melanoma (without discernable pigment)* may be very
difficult.
(Papanicolaou stain, x600).

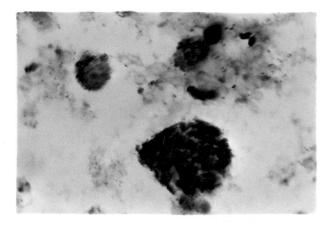

Fig. 7.27
For comparison with the previous slide, this slide shows
the picture of a fine-needle aspirate from *lymph node
metastasis from pigmented malignant melanoma*. The
background is necrotic.
(Papanicolaou stain, x600).

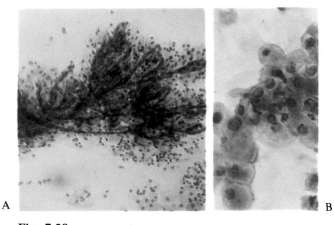

A   B

Fig. 7.28
Fine-needle aspirate from a cervical lymph node.
A: Metastatic epithelial cells arranged in solid strands
with a rich vascular component. In M.G.G. preparations,
the cytoplasm appears larger, clear or slightly basophilic.
B: The metastatic cells, at a higher magnification: they
are round-shaped, with a small nucleus, sometimes
peripherically situated; note the clear and granular gray
areas, in the cytoplasm.
A diagnosis of *lymph node metastasis from renal,
clear-cell carcinoma (granular type)* was made. Intrave-
nous pyelography showed distorsion of the parenchymal
pattern caused by a mass in the left kydney.
(A: M.G.G. stain, x63; B: Papanicolaou stain, x250).

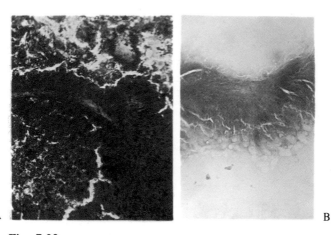

A   B

Fig. 7.29
The same case as in the previous slide.
A: The metastatic cells are highly positive to periodic
acid-Schiff stain.
B: The positivity to periodic acid-Schiff stain is due to
glycogen, and therefore it is not resistant to diastase
digestion. The red magenta stain persists in the collagen;
peripherically the cytoplasm of the metastatic cells
appears as a colorless, round structure.
(A: PAS stain, x63; B: PAS stain after diastase digestion,
x63).

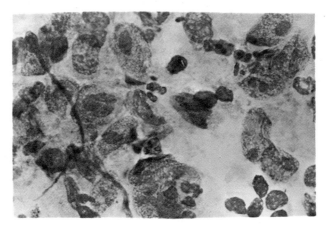

Fig. 7.30
Fine-needle aspirate from a cervical lymph node; note
metastatic cells, with decreased cohesion, ovoid or
irregular in shape; the nuclei are large, often round with
a very prominent nucleolus (inclusion body-like). A
diagnosis of possible *lymph node metastasis from naso-
pharynx carcinoma* was made (histologically confirmed).
Similar pictures, if binucleated cells (Reed-Sternberg-like)
are present and intermingled with large numbers of
eosinophils, may sometimes be erroneously diagnosed as
Hodgkin's lymphoma.
(M.G.G. stain, x630).

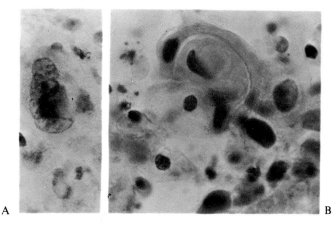

A   B

Fig. 7.31
Fine-needle aspirate from a subclavian "cyst". Approximately 10 ml of yellow, fairly clear fluid were withdrawn, filtered through Millipore[⊕] and the collected cells transferred onto a frozen slide (according to a modified filter imprint technique).
The features shown in A and B correspond to an epithelial malignancy. A diagnosis of ***metastasis (which had undergone liquefaction) from a well-differentiated epidermoid carcinoma*** was made (see, in B, concentric pearl-like structure). The origin of the metastatic cells was a primary lung neoplasm.
(A, B: Papanicolaou stain, x630).

8
BREAST

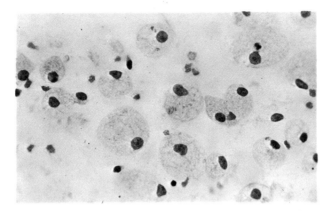

Fig. 8.1
Fine-needle aspirate from a hard breast lump. This lesion was really a *cyst* from which approximately 10 ml of turbid fluid were withdrawn. Monomorphic pattern of benign, quite isometric, round foamy cells (spongiocytes), with small peripheral nuclei, which sometimes contain nucleoli.
Sometimes, these cells do not show macrophagic activity, even in a hemorrhagic fluid, whereas, at other times, they phagocytize iron pigment: therefore, it is likely that some spongiocytes are of epithelial origin, whereas others are of histiocytic origin.
(Filter imprint technique modified, Papanicolaou stain, x630).

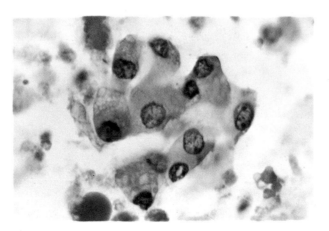

Fig. 8.2
Material aspirated from a *breast cyst*; cluster of apocrine cells ("oncocytes", "cells in sweat metaplasia") showing round or ovoid nuclei (sometimes with nucleoli), with an even thickening of the membrane; the cytoplasm is large, highly eosinophilic, either homogeneous or foamy.
(Cytocentrifuge, Papanicolaou stain, x600).

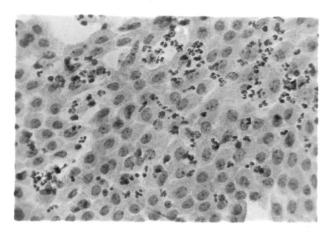

Fig. 8.3
Apocrine sheet, aspirated from breast cyst, demonstrating
acute superimposed inflammation (numerous neutrophils
can be seen).
(Papanicolaou stain, x63).

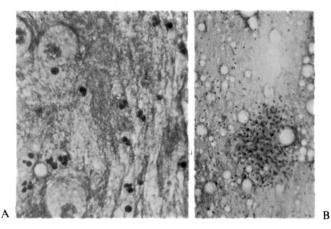

Fig. 8.4
Fine-needle aspirate from a hard non-mobile breast lump,
with irregular edges, highly suggestive of malignancy, on
physical examination.
A: Mononucleated histiocytes, mixed with neutrophils
and necrotic debris.
B: Fibroblasts involved in the repair process; the
background is composed of adipocytes.
Diagnosis of *fat necrosis* was made (favourable outcome).
(A: M.G.G. stain, x630, B: Papanicolaou stain, x125).

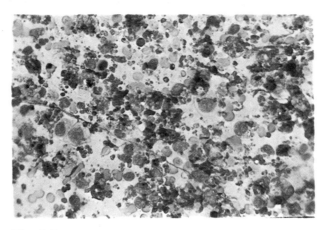

Fig. 8.5
Fine-needle aspirate of a palpable post-traumatic breast
lump; the cells are mainly histiocytes; many of them have
phagocytized hemosiderin, represented by coarse, black
granules within a cytoplasm containing small vacuoles.
Diagnosis of a ***previously contused lesion (with an
important hemorrhagic component)*** was made.
Favourable outcome.
(M.G.G. stain, x240).

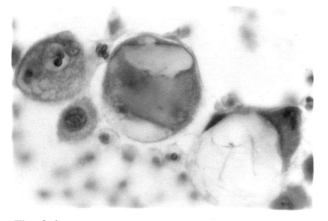

Fig. 8.6
Fine-needle aspirate of a palpable breast lump *(paraffino-
ma)*; one can observe large histiocytes, with nucleoli and
large cytoplasmic vacuoles.
(Papanicolaou stain, x600).

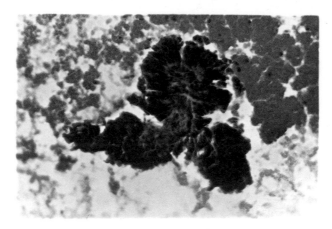

Fig. 8.7
Fragment of a papillomatous structure, observed in a specimen of fluid, obtained by fine-needle aspiration from a breast cyst: the papillae show a collagen-vascular core, covered with a multilayered columnar epithelium. The background is hemorrhagic. (Tissue section diagnosis: *endocystic papilloma*).
(Papanicolaou stain, x250).

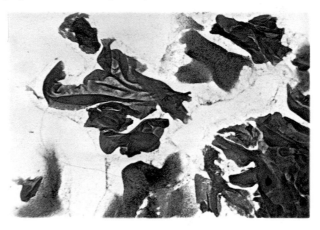

Fig. 8.8
Fine-needle aspirate of a mobile, palpable, breast lump: highly cellular field, made up of sheets (sometimes folded) of benign ductal epithelium, fibrocollagen stromal fragments and naked bipolar nuclei (cytological diagnosis: *fibroadenoma*).
(Papanicolaou stain, x30).

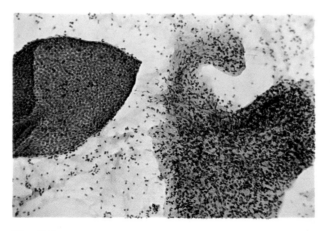

Fig. 8.9
The cytological diagnosis of *fibroadenoma* can only be
made (at medium magnification) when the following three
structures are present: sheets of ductal epithelium,
background of naked bipolar nuclei and fibrocollagen
fragments.
(Papanicolaou stain, x250).

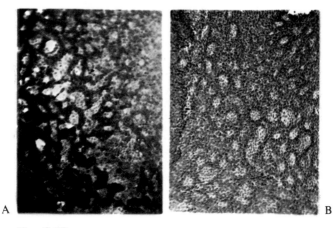

A   B

Fig. 8.10
In aspirates from *fibroadenomatous lesions with a florid
epithelial component*, the ductal sheets sometimes appear
strangely "crumpled", with a pseudo-cribriform appearance. This is to be differentiated from the cribriform
aspect of intraductal carcinoma (see Figs. 8.21 and 8.22)
(A: M.G.G. stain, x63; B: Papanicolaou stain, x63).

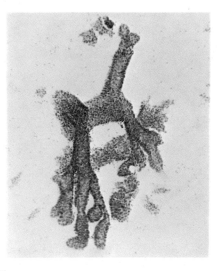

Fig. 8.11
Fine-needle aspirate from a small breast lump, with
indistinct edges: benign ductal and apocrine sheets, a few
naked bipolar nuclei (not visible at this magnification).
In this case, because no stromal component was seen, a
***non-malignant lesion (possibly fibroadenoma-fibroadeno-
sis)*** was diagnosed.
(Papanicolaou stain, x63).

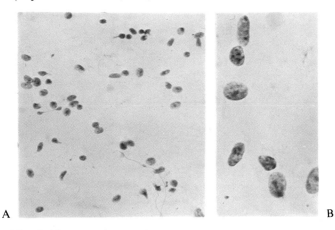

A   B

Fig. 8.12
Fine-needle aspirate from a breast ***fibroadenoma***. In this
case only naked bipolar nuclei (probably derived from
the myoepithelial ductal cells) can be observed; these are
peculiarly fragile and lose their cytoplasm because of the
traumatic effect of aspiration.
Such nuclei are usually oval-shaped, often demonstrate
a nucleolus and even thickening of the membrane.
(A: Papanicolaou stain, x63; B: Papanicolaou stain, x400).

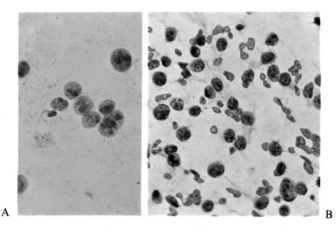

A   B

Fig. 8.13
A: Fine-needle aspirate from breast *fibroadenoma*. The
naked bipolar nuclei have, especially during pregnancy
and lactation, a round rather than oval shape and
prominent nucleoli; in this case, they are to be differentiated from malignant, naked nuclei.
B: Malignant hyperchromatic naked nuclei, with marked
anisonucleosis. The background is necrotic.
(A: Papanicolaou stain, x400, B: Papanicolaou stain,
x240).

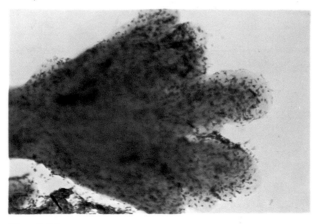

Fig. 8.14
Fine-needle aspirate from breast *fibroadenoma* (elsewhere
in the slide, naked bipolar nuclei and epithelial sheets).
The club-like structure indicates the intracanalicular type.
(Papanicolaou stain, x250).

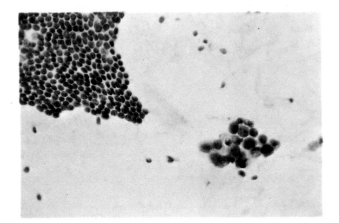

Fig. 8.15
Fine-needle aspirate of a palpable, breast lump, consisting
of a soft, parenchymatous area (tissue section diagnosis:
ductal, infiltrating carcinoma n.o.s.) next to an area of
a highly increased consistency (tissue section diagnosis:
sclerosing adenosis). The material collected by the
fine-needle represents the result of a "mixed" sampling,
derived from the two lesions. One can observe an
epithelial benign sheet (top, left) and naked bipolar nuclei
(derived from the adenosis) next to a cluster of obviously
malignant cells (bottom, right). In this case, therefore, the
naked bipolar nuclei are present in a slide showing
malignancy; this is rarely observed and by itself does not
contradict the general principle according to which the
presence of naked bipolar nuclei is almost always
indicative of a non-malignant lesion. In the above case,
the mixed sampling results in an obviously malignant
cytological picture, characterized by the simultaneous
presence of malignant cells and naked bipolar nuclei.
(Papanicolaou stain, x250).

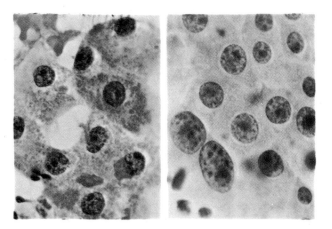

Fig. 8.16
Fine-needle aspirate from a palpable, breast lump (elswhere in the slide, the picture suggests fibroadenoma). The slide shows two fields of the lesion characterized by *apocrine metaplasia* with a marked anisonucleosis. The nuclear hypertrophy is accompanied by an increase in the cytoplasmic area (and therefore the nuclear-cytoplasmic ratio is not modified). Such a picture of highly marked anisonucleosis is compatible with a *non-malignant apocrine metaplasia*.
(Papanicolaou stain, x630).

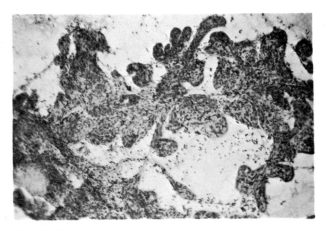

Fig. 8.17
Fine-needle aspirate performed ten days after delivery. One can observe a benign structure, lobular-type, formed by enlarged acini, with a large number of naked bipolar nuclei.
(Papanicolaou stain, x63).

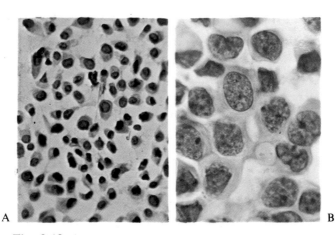

Fig. 8.18
A: Fine-needle aspirate from a breast neoplasm: the slide is highly cellular with a monomorphic pattern (this picture is usually, but not always, observed in malignant lesions).
B: The same case, at a higher magnification. The *epithelial malignant cells* are in part cohesive (the malignant cells are isolated to a great extent in the more-dedifferentiated neoplasm, because of their reduced cohesiveness); the nuclei are irregular-shaped; one can observe some anisonucleosis, coarse chromatin and irregular thickening of the membranes. Prominent eosinophilic nucleoli are sometimes seen.
(A: Papanicolaou stain, x125; B: Papanicolaou stain, x400).

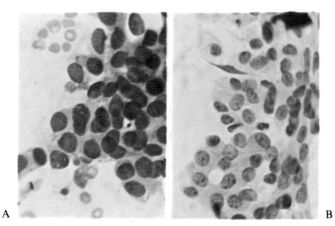

A   B

Fig. 8.19
Cytological picture of a *highly-differentiated, breast adenocarcinoma:* cohesive sheets of rectangular cells, with round nuclei and the sharp-edged cytoplasm displaced to one side. This picture, which does not present remarkable atypias, can be mistakenly considered benign (in breast cytology, the false negatives, or false benigns, constitute approximately 10% of the various series reported; these may be due either to undervaluation of highly-differentiated neoplasms or to samplings made outside the malignant area, in complex lesions). It should be noted that, in well-differentiated breast cancers, the nuclear-cytoplasmic ratio appears paradoxically more favourable than in the benign ductal cells of a fibroadenoma, since the cytoplasmic area is increased, showing a peculiar secretory polarity.
(A: M.G.G. stain, x125; B: Papanicolaou stain, x125).

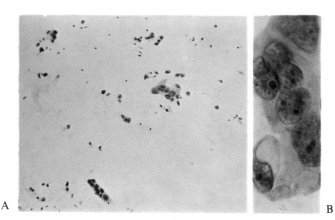

A   B

Fig. 8.20
A: Fine-needle aspirate from a palpable breast lump; the
slide is hypocellular (compare with Figure 8.18), but the
cytological picture is obviously malignant; the collected
material corresponds to an effectively satisfactory
sampling from a *highly sclerotic carcinoma* (in these cases,
the rule "malignancy = extremely cellular slides" is not
proved; furthermore, it is to be remembered that highly
cellular slides are often the rule in benign lesions, such
as fibroadenomas).
B: Malignant epithelial cells, at a higher magnification,
showing anisonucleosis, overlapping of the nuclei, coarse
chromatin and prominent nucleoli.
(A: Papanicolaou stain, x63; B: Papanicolaou stain, x630).

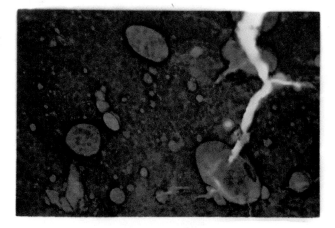

Fig. 8.21
Epithelial fragment aspirated from a palpable, breast
lump: the cytological three-dimensional picture suggests
the *cribriform pattern of intraductal carcinoma*.
(Papanicolaou stain, x125).

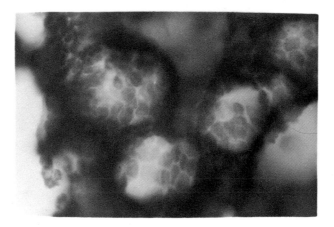

Fig. 8.22
A case similar to the previous one, at a higher
magnification: the cribriform aspect is made up of hollow,
round spaces in an intraductal neoplasia (compare this
three-dimensional fragment with the crumpled ductal
sheets obtained from a fibroadenoma, in Figure 8.12).
(Papanicolaou stain, x250).

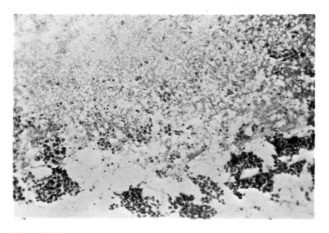

Fig. 8.23
Fine-needle aspirate from a palpable breast lump: clusters
of malignant epithelial cells seem to surround some
necrotic material; diagnosis of ***intraductal carcinoma*** was
made (tissue-section diagnosis: ***comedocarcinoma***). It is
unusual to find necrotic material in infiltrating tumors;
in intraductal carcinoma, the morphology of the neoplastic cells is undistinguishable from that of infiltrating
types.
(Papanicolaou stain, x63).

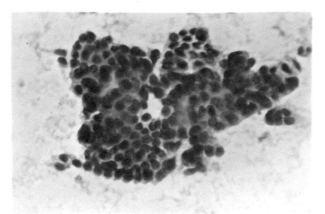

Fig. 8.24
Fine-needle aspirate of a palpable breast lump: *malignant epithelial sheet* (tissue section diagnosis: *ductal carcinoma n.o.s.*). The nuclei are hyperchromatic, cleaved, sometimes unevenly superposed, especially at the periphery of the sheet.
Naked bipolar nuclei are not present; on a necrotic background, detached neoplastic cells can be observed.
(Papanicolaou stain, x250).

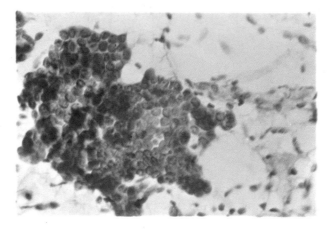

Fig. 8.25
Note, for comparison, at the same magnification, a ductal sheet from a *fibroadenoma*. The nuclei present a pale chromatinic network, do not demonstrate atypias and appear monolayered at the edges of the sheet.
Numerous naked nuclei are present together with an amorphous, myxoid stromal-like material.
(Papanicolaou stain, x250).

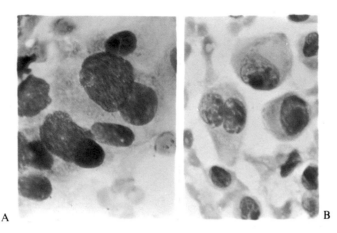

A   B

Fig. 8.26
In A, a fine-needle aspirate from a palpable breast lump:
ductal infiltrating carcinoma n.o.s., large cell-type,
corresponding to a partially cohesive sheet of malignant
cells, sometimes large and with superposition; these are
characterized by marked anisonucleosis and prominent
nucleoli.
In B, a lesion similar to the previous one. Remarkable
anisocytosis of malignant epithelial cells, which are
hyperchromatic, generally large, sometimes with two
nuclei; the chromatin is coarse, the nuclear membranes
are thickened and the nucleoli prominent.
(A: M.G.G. stain, x600; B: Papanicolaou stain, x600).

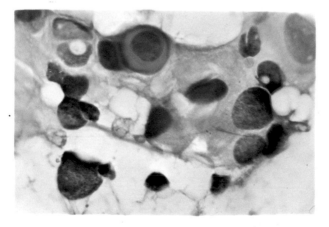

Fig. 8.27
Fine-needle aspirate from a breast ***carcinoma n.o.s., large
cell-type***. The orangeophilic cell indicates an epidermoidal metaplasia.
(Papanicolaou stain, x600).

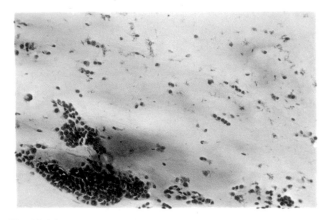

Fig. 8.28
Fine-needle aspirate from a palpable breast lump: clusters
of malignant epithelial cells interspersed with stripes of
amorphous gray-greenish material (mucus). Diagnosis of
colloid carcinoma was made (tissue section diagnosis:
colloid carcinoma).
(Papanicolaou stain, x63).

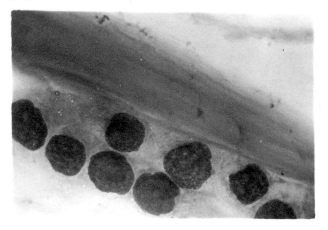

Fig. 8.29
Fine-needle aspirate from a lesion histologically similar
to the previous one. Note the fibrillar aspect of the stripes
of mucus which are red-stained and the slight atypia of
the epithelial malignant cells.
(M.G.G. stain, x600).

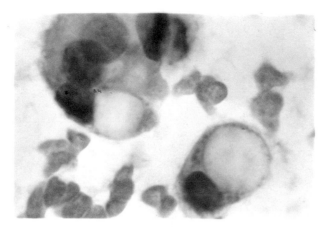

Fig. 8.30
Fine-needle aspirate from a ***mucin-producing carcinoma
of the breast, signet-ring cell type***. In this tumor,
extracellular mucin is scanty (unlike in the more frequent
colloid carcinoma). The differentiation between colloid
and signet-ring carcinoma is very important from a
practical point of view; the latter has a more severe
prognosis than colloid carcinoma, which has a less-
aggressive natural history, less common axillary lymph
metastates and prolonged survival.
Mucin stain should be done routinely, on all breast
carcinomas where numerous vacuolated cells are present;
vacuoles in some neoplastic cells may sometimes represent degenerative products or secretory lipids, such as
that seen in so-called lipid-rich carcinomas.
(Papanicolaou stain, x600).

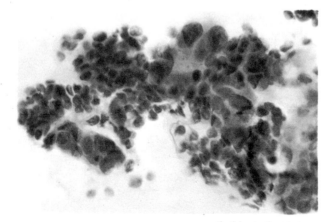

Fig. 8.31
Fine-needle aspirate from a palpable breast lump:
malignant cluster suggesting a ***poorly differentiated apocrine carcinoma***. The nuclei are hyperchromatic, polymorphous, crowded, with irregular superposition. The
cytoplasm of some malignant cells is large, eosinophilic,
finely granulated, with features suggesting apocrine
metaplasia.
(Papanicolaou stain, x250).

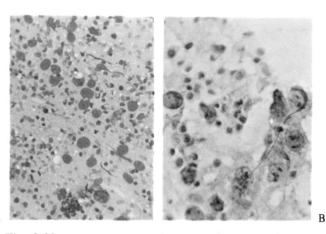

A   B

Fig. 8.32
A: Fine-needle aspirate from a palpable breast lump. One
can observe fairly large, malignant cells; the nuclei are
round or ovoid, sometimes naked. There is marked
anisonucleosis. These cells are intermingled with a rich
lymphocytic component. Diagnosis of *medullary carcino-*
ma was made. (This tumor is also called *acinic cell*
carcinoma because of the similarity between these
neoplastic cells and the benign cells surrounding the
lumina of the acini of the lactating breast).
B: Cytologic picture of a fine-needle aspirate from a lesion
similar to that in A: marked anaplastic, epithelial
malignant cells and necrosis; very rich lymphocytic
component.
(A: M.G.G. stain, x125; B: Papanicolaou stain, x250).

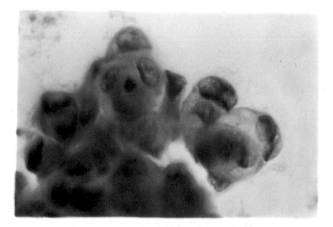

Fig. 8.33
This slide was prepared with a fluid aspirated, using a
fine-needle, from a cystic lesion of the breast; one can
observe a malignant papillary structure, formed by
atypical, multilayered hyperchromatic cells. Diagnosis of
papillary-cystic carcinoma was made (tissue section
diagnosis: *papillary-cystic carcinoma*).
(Cytocentrifuge, Papanicolaou stain, x600).

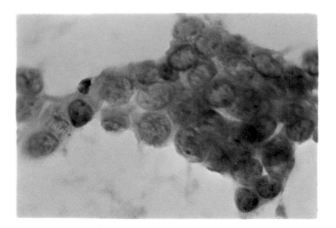

Fig. 8.34
Fine-needle aspirate from a palpable breast lump: the
malignant sheet consists of monomorphous round-shaped
cells, which are sometimes superposed and characterised
by an increase in the nuclear-cytoplasmic ratio and
irregular thickening of the nuclear membrane. Naked
bipolar nuclei are absent.
Such a picture represents the cytological counterpart of
the so-called *tubular carcinoma* (low-grade malignancy).
(Papanicolaou stain, x600).

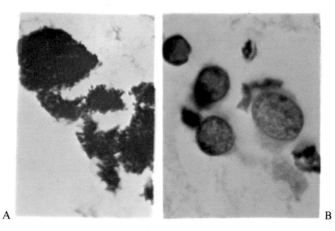

A   B

Fig. 8.35
A: In this fine-needle aspirate, clusters are represented,
resembling the structure of the distal intralobular ducts.
The clusters are formed by monomorphic, crowded,
superposed cells. This picture corresponds to a *lobular
carcinoma in situ.*
B: *Lobular carcinoma in situ:* note single isolated cells,
which constitute a fairly monomorphous population; the
nuclear-cytoplasmic ratio is highly increased, the chromatin is coarse and the nuclear membrane demonstrates
marked thickening.
(A: Papanicolaou stain, x125; B: Papanicolaou stain,
x1250).

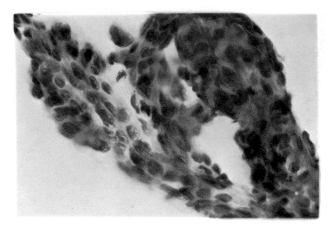

Fig. 8.36
In *florid fibroadenomatosis of the male breast,* the
hyperplastic ductal sheets sometimes demonstrate three-
dimensional aspects and irregular polarity of the cells,
which are often hyperchromatic and of different sizes.
Moreover the naked nuclei are sometimes missing and
the final diagnosis requires a tissue section procedure.
(Papanicolaou stain, x250).

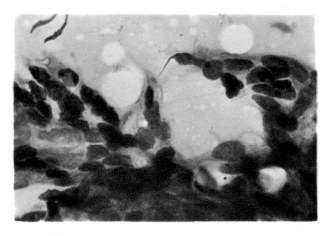

Fig. 8.37
Fine-needle aspirate from a large breast lump, clinically
defined as *"phyllodes tumor".* The collected material
suggests a highly cellular sarcomatous component with
fairly polymorphous and sometimes superposed cells
arranged in a parallel fashion.
(M.G.G. stain, x125).

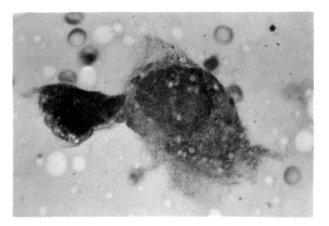

Fig. 8.38
The same case as in the previous slide. Note, at a higher magnification, huge, bizarre, extremely polymorphic sarcomatous cells (tissue section diagnosis: ***cystosarcoma phyllodes***).
(M.G.G. stain, x600).

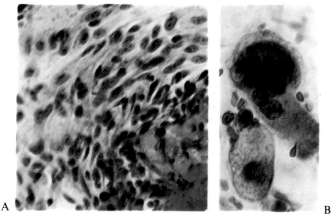

A   B

Fig. 8.39
Fine-needle aspirate from a palpable breast mass: approximately 1 ml of yellow, viscid, foamy fluid was withdrawn (similar to that usually obtained from lesions due to fat necrosis). The spindle cells arranged in parallel fashion (in A) were erroneously judged to be fibroblasts involved in a repair process; the multinucleated, giant cells with foamy cytoplasm (in B) were believed to be histiocytes from a foreign body reaction.
However, the tissue diagnosis was of ***breast carcinoma, with extremely metaplastic spindle cells (pseudofibroblast cells), osteoklast-like cells and cartilagineous metaplasia.***
Re-examination of the cytological smears failed to demonstrate any cartilagineous, aspirate structure.
(A: Papanicolaou stain, x250; B: Papanicolaou stain, x630).

9
MEDIASTINUM

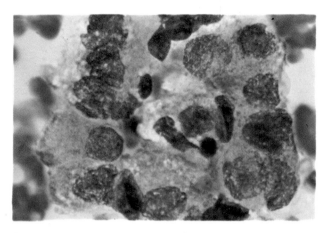

Fig. 9.1
Fine-needle aspirate from a mediastinal mass. Note clustered malignant epithelial cells, exhibiting fairly large nuclei with membrane folds, occasional prominent nucleoli, pale blue-stained cytoplasm with microvacuoles. A generic diagnosis of *malignancy (possibly epithelial)* was made (the tissue section diagnosis was of *embryonal carcinoma*, probably primary in the mediastinum). (M.G.G. stain, x600).

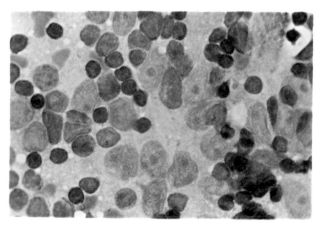

Fig. 9.2
Fine-needle aspirate from a paramediastinal mass, performed percutaneously. Innumerable lymphoid cells intermingled with less-numerous, larger (epithelial) cells; the latter show cyanophilic cytoplasm with indistinct boundaries, and roundish or ovoid, hypochromatic nuclei and evident, mostly central, round nucleoli. A diagnosis of *thymoma, prevalently lymphocytic,* was made (histologically confirmed). (M.G.G. stain, x600).

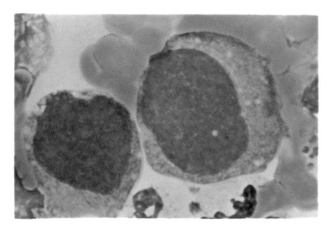

Fig. 9.3
Fine-needle aspirate from a mediastinal mass. Two
malignant, irregularly roundish-shaped cells, with well-
defined edges are depicted.
The nuclei are large and the nuclear membranes sharp
(especially in Papanicolaou preparations); the nucleoli
appear indistinct. Elsewhere in the slides prepared, these
cells are characteristically monolayered.
This picture suggests ***seminoma, primary in the mediastinum*** (the cytologic diagnosis was histologically confirmed).
(M.G.G. stain, x1250).

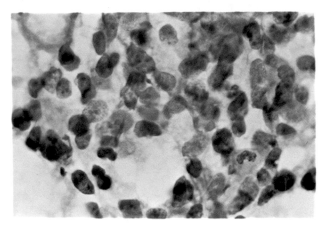

Fig. 9.4
Fine-needle aspirate from a mediastinal mass. Neoplastic,
small, monomorphic cells, which appear haphazardly
overlapping, with hyperchromatic, irregular nuclei; the
nuclear membranes are thickened and the nucleoli
prominent. Note (left) a characteristic, rosette-like, cellular arrangement. A diagnosis of ***neuroblastoma*** was made
(histologically confirmed).
(Papanicolaou stain, x125).

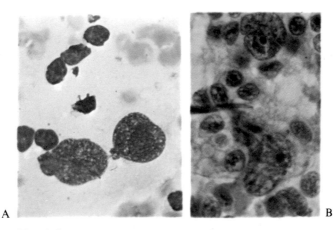

A   B

Fig. 9.5
Fine-needle aspirate from a mediastinal mass, performed
percutaneously using a parasternal approach. In A and
B, Reed-Sternberg cells are depicted (elsewhere in the
slides prepared, eosinophilis, lymphocytes and mononu-
cleated Hodgkin's cells were present). A diagnosis of
Hodgkin's lymphoma , nodular sclerosing type, was made.
(A: M.G.G. stain, x600; B: Papanicolaou stain, x600).

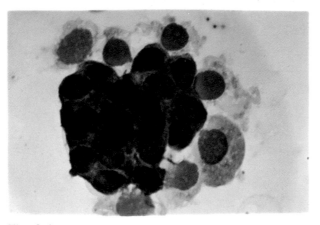

Fig. 9.6
Fine-needle aspirate from a mediastinal mass, performed
percutaneously with parasternal approach and fluoroscopic guidance. Approximately 10 ml of yellow fluid were
withdrawn.
A sheet of mesothelial cells is depicted. A diagnosis of
pericardial cyst was made.
(Cytocentrifuge, M.G.G. stain, x250).

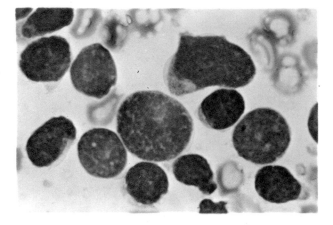

Fig. 9.7
Fine-needle aspirate from mediastinal mass. Malignant
"lymphoid" cells, fairly irregular in shape and size are
depicted. Note the occasional multiple nucleoli.
A diagnosis of *lymphoblastic lymphoma* was made.
(M.G.G. stain, x600).

10
LUNG

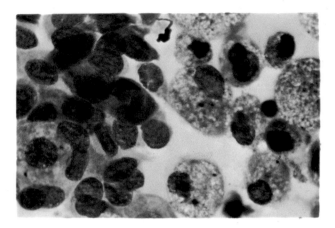

Fig. 10.1
Fine-needle aspirate from a normal lung: note epithelial
cuboid cells from terminal bronchioles, intermingled with
carbon-particle-laden macrophages.
(M.G.G. stain, x600).

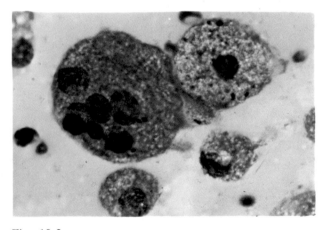

Fig. 10.2
The same case as in the previous slide. The macrophages
are variable-sized and sometimes multinucleated.
(M.G.G. stain, x600).

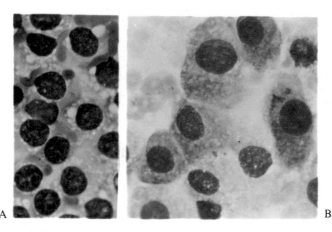

A   B

Fig. 10.3
A: Fine-needle aspirate from a pulmonary nodule.
Roentgenograms revealed diffuse infiltrates in both lungs,
interpreted as prolonged inflammatory disease. These
benign cells were classified as *"pneumocytes"* because of
their characteristic honeycomb arrangement. The outcome was favourable.
B: Isolated pneumocytes, at a higher magnification. The
cells from the terminal bronchioles are cuboid or
polyhedral; the nuclei are ovoid and the cytoplasm large
with sharp edges.
(M.G.G. stain, A: x250; B: x600).

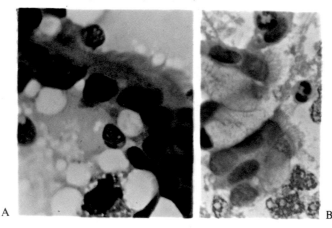

A   B

Fig. 10.4
A: ***Sheet of bronchial epithelium***, obtained with fine-
needle aspiration. Note well-preserved cilia of the
columnar cells, which are next to a carbon-particle-laden
macrophage.
B: With fine-needle aspiration, columnar ciliated cells,
red blood cells and one neutrophil have been collected.
(A: M.G.G. stain, x250; B: Papanicolaou stain, x250).

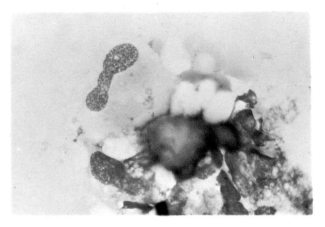

Fig. 10.5
Fine-needle aspirate from a peripheral pulmonary nodule:
note, in the midfield, a calcified roundshaped structure
surrounded by cells, some of which are classifiable as
epithelioid. The very characteristic, elongated nuclear
shapes are due to aspiration trauma and not to the
preparation of the slide (these features, in fact, are never
observed in imprint preparations). In similar cases, the
cytological diagnosis of **_possible tuberculosis_** must be
proved by culture of _Mycobacterium tuberculosis_ from
the aspirate.
(M.G.G. stain, x600).

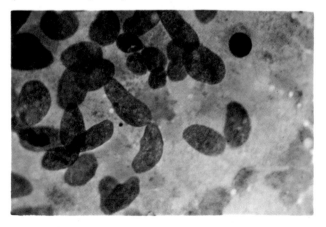

Fig. 10.6
Lung aspirate from which _Mycobacterium tuberculosis_
was cultured. Note Langhans' multinucleated giant cell.
(M.G.G. stain, x600).

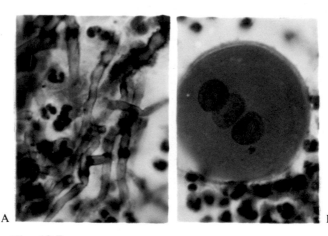

A   B

Fig. 10.7
Aspirate from a ***pulmonary aspergilloma*** (direct smear):
A: Note branching septate hyphae, intermingled with
neutrophils.
B: Severe atypia in the cell, demonstrating epidermoidal
metaplasia (note three nuclei and two-tone cytoplasm).
(A and B: Papanicolaou stain, x600).

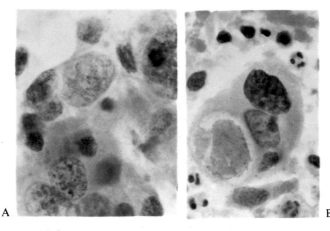

A   B

Fig. 10.8
Aspirate from a ***fairly well-differentiated epidermoid
carcinoma of the lung***. Note, in A and B, pleomorphic
neoplastic cells, some of which are keratinized (B);
necrosis in the background.
(A, B: Papanicolaou stain, x600).

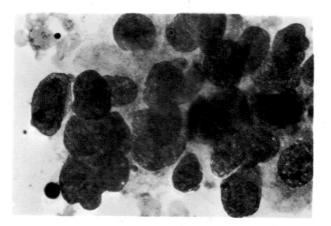

Fig. 10.9
Aspirate from a ***moderately-differentiated lung adenocarcinoma***; note cluster of fairly monomorphic malignant cells which demonstrate little cytoplasm and evident nucleoli.
(M.G.G. stain, x600).

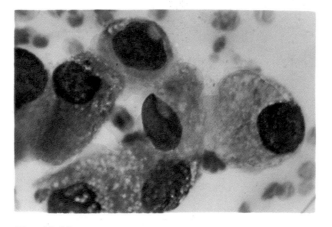

Fig. 10.10
Aspirate from a ***poorly-differentiated lung adenocarcinoma***. Note malignant isolated cells, anisonucleosis, cytoplasmic microvacuoles and small nucleoli.
(M.G.G. stain, x600).

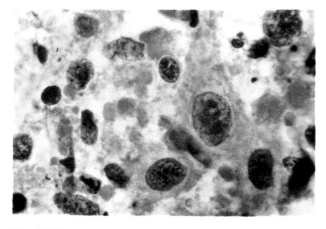

Fig. 10.11
Fine-needle aspirate from a *lung carcinoma, classifiable as anaplastic, large-cell type:* note necrotic background and pleomorphic malignant cells, some of which are large. Keratinization is absent.
(Papanicolaou stain, x600).

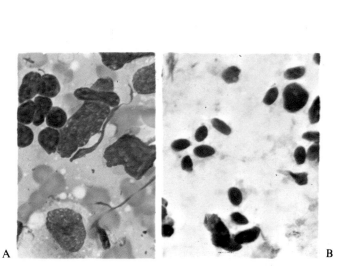

A   B

Fig. 10.12
Fine-needle aspirate from *anaplastic, small-cell type lung carcinoma*.
A: The malignant cells, which are reduced to naked nuclei, appear crowded.
B: Moderate anisonucleosis in the malignant cells; note some "oat"-like nuclei and nuclear moulding (bottom).
(A: M.G.G. stain, x600; B: Papanicolaou stain, x600).

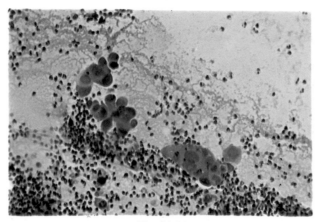

Fig. 10.13

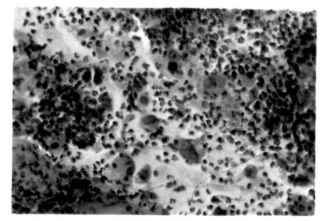

Fig. 10.14

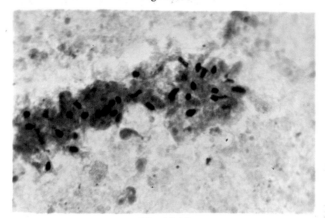

Fig. 10.15

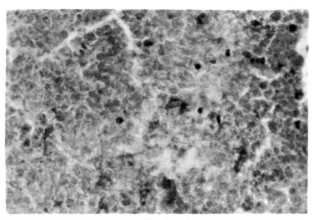

Fig. 10.16

Figs. 10.13, 10.14, 10.15 and 10.16
Fine-needle aspirates from peripheral pulmonary nodules,
diagnosed as *epidermoid carcinomas*. The cells depicted
in Figure 10.13 are derived from the more peripheral,
better-nourished part of the neoplasm, where the prolife-
rative activity is more marked than differentiation: the
general features are more suggestive of adenocarcinoma
than epidermoid neoplasm. The material depicted in
Figure 10.14 was aspirated from the central, poorly-
nourished, more differentiated and partially necrotic part
of the same neoplasm. The cytological picture is without
doubt that of an epidermoid carcinoma, but because of
the necrosis, the general features are more like those of
a sputum specimen preparation than a fine-needle
aspirate, in which the cells are collected in a living state,
as in bronchial brush specimens, and, therefore, usually
well-preserved. The features depicted in Figures 10.15
and 10.16 were observed in material collected by
transcutaneous fine-needle aspiration from other cases of
epidermoid carcinoma of the lung. The material aspirated
is largely necrotic and one can only note very rare,
malignant, epidermoidal cells.
(Fig. 10.13: Papanicolaou stain, x125; Figs. 10.14, 10.15
and 10.16: Papanicolaou stain, x250).

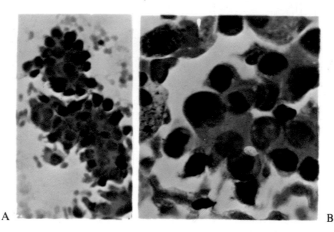

A   B

Fig. 10.17
Note in A and B, *clusters of adenocarcinomatous cells*
obtained from a peripheral lung nodule, by percutaneous
fine-needle aspiration. The cytoplasmic eosinophilia is
probably due to drying because of delayed fixation of the
spread material; this picture may lead to an incorrect
diagnosis of epidermoid carcinoma. The adenocarcinomatous nature of the neoplasm is suggested by the obvious
papillary structure and some aspects of secretive polarity.
(A: Papanicolaou stain, x250; B: Papanicolaou stain,
x600).

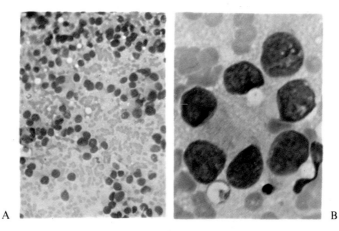

A   B

Fig. 10.18
Fine-needle aspirate from a *bronchoalveolar carcinoma*:
note, in A and B, characteristically ring-patterned
malignant cells, reproducing alveolar structures.
(A: M.G.G. stain, x100; B: M.G.G. stain, x600).

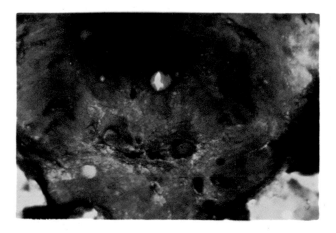

Fig. 10.19
Fine-needle aspirate from a peripheral lung nodule, which
showed sharp edges roentgenologically (during needling, a
hard consistency was noticed.) The aspirated material is
cartilage: note densely basophilic condrocytes· in a
red-purple ground substance.
A diagnosis of *hamartochondroma* was made (histologically confirmed).
(M.G.G. stain, x125).

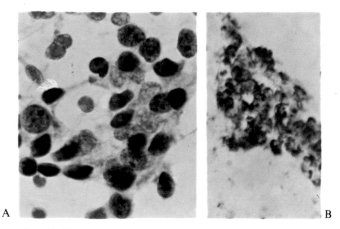

A   B

Fig. 10.20
A: Fine-needle aspirate from a peripheral lung nodule: a
fairly monomorphic population of small neoplastic
slightly atypical cells can be observed.
B: note the many neurosecretory cytoplasmic granules.
A cytological diagnosis of *carcinoid tumor* was made
(histologically confirmed).
(A: Papanicolaou stain, x400; B: Grimelius, x125).

11
LIVER

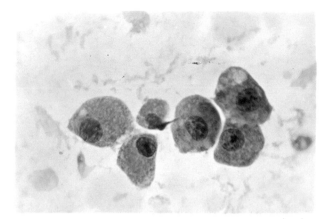

Fig.11.1
Normal hepatocytes in a fine-needle aspirate from a
palpable liver mass. The cells are polyhedral with sharp
boundaries; the nuclei show slight variability in size, the
nucleoli are evident and the cytoplasm displays reddish
granules.
(Papanicolaou stain, x600).

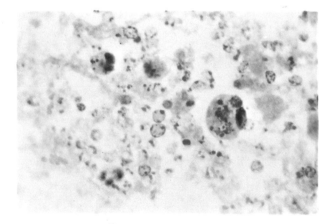

Fig. 11.2
This preparation was made with smeared fluid, withdrawn
with a fine-needle from a *hepatic pseudocyst*: note bloody
background and histiocytes.
(Papanicolaou stain, x600).

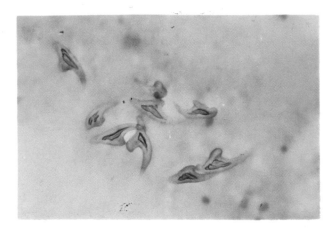

Fig. 11.3
This preparation was made with some clear, yellow fluid
withdrawn from a hepatic "cyst". Note the numerous,
characteristic hooklets. A diagnosis of ***Echinococcus cyst***
was made.
(Cytocentrifuge, M.G.G. stain, x600).

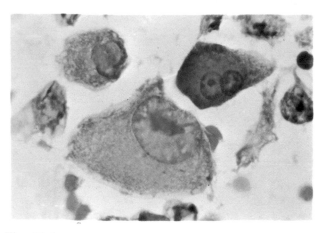

Fig. 11.4
Percutaneous aspirate of a palpable hepatic mass: note
non-cohesive, large, liver cells (for comparison see Fig.
11.1); there is marked anisocytosis. The nuclei are
sometimes multiple and characterised by irregular
thickening of the membranes and bounding clumped
chromatin. In the midfield, there is a cell with an irregular
macronucleolus. A diagnosis of ***hepatocellular carcinoma***
was made.
(Papanicolaou stain, x600).

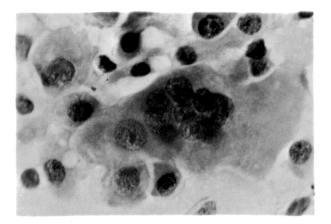

Fig. 11.5
Percutaneous, fine-needle aspirate from a palpable hepatic mass. *Hepatocellular carcinoma cells* are depicted. They show marked anisocytosis and obviously malignant nuclear characteristics; in the midfield, a huge, multinucleate cell is also present.
(Papanicolaou stain, x600).

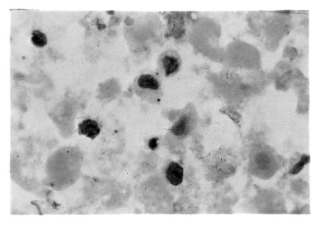

Fig. 11.6
Percutaneous, fine-needle aspirate from a hepatic mass, performed under ultrasonic guidance. Note necrotic debris, shadow cells and sparse, epidermoid cells, still fairly well-preserved. A diagnosis of *liver metastasis of epidermoid carcinoma* was made.
(Papanicolaou stain, x600).

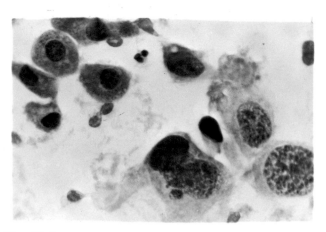

Fig. 11.7
Percutaneous, fine-needle aspirate from a hepatic mass,
performed under ultrasonic guidance.
Note (lower-right corner) malignant cells, probably from
a *moderately-differentiated epidermoid carcinoma* (for
comparison see normal hepatocytes in the upper-left
corner of the slide).
(Papanicolaou stain, x600).

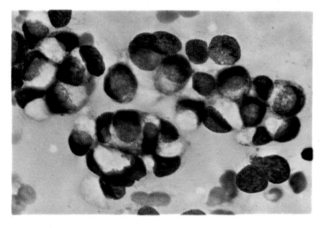

Fig. 11.8
Percutaneous, fine-needle aspirate performed under ultrasonic guidance. Note clusters of malignant, signet-ring
cells. A diagnosis of *liver metastasis of mucosecreting
adenocarcinoma* was made (primary in the stomach).
(M.G.G. stain, x600).

12
PANCREAS

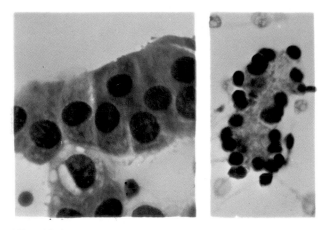

Fig. 12.1
Cells aspirated from a ***normal pancreatic area***. Note ductal
epithelium (A, seen from above) and the acinic structure
(B). The cells from the main ducts are tall and columnar;
the acinic cells are pyramid-shaped, with small hyperchromatic nuclei and cyanophilic, granular cytoplasm.
(A: M.G.G. stain, x600; B: Papanicolaou stain, x600).

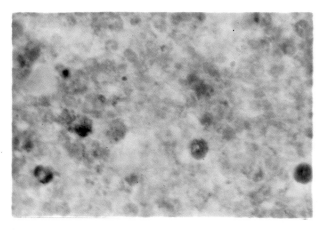

Fig. 12.2
Fine-needle aspirate taken percutaneously from a ***pancreatic pseudocyst***, under ultrasonic guidance: necrotic
debris, some lysed, red blood cells and a few neutrophils.
(Papanicolaou stain, x600).

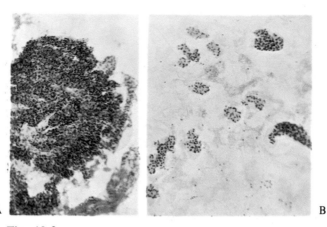

A   B

Fig. 12.3
Fine-needle aspirate (at laparotomy) from a hard mass
in the pancreatic head (clinically suspected of malignancy).
In A, acini intermingled with fibrous tissue; in B,
dissociated acinar structures, necrotic background. There
is no evidence of malignancy. A diagnosis of *chronic
sclerosing pancreatitis* was made. In a three-year follow-
up, there was no evidence of malignant disease.
(A: Papanicolaou stain, x125; B: Papanicolaou stain,
x125).

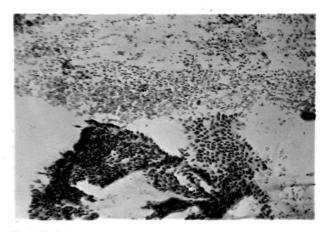

Fig. 12.4
Fine-needle aspirate (at laparotomy) from a mass in the
pancreatic head (clinically suspected of malignancy). In
the upper-half of the slide, the picture is suggestive of
pancreatitis (inflammatory and necrotic cells); in the
lower-half, clusters of malignant cells *(moderately differentiated adenocarcinoma)*.
Fine-needle aspiration allows deep, multiple sampling
from malignant lesions, below the peripheral zone of
pancreatitis. In cases where the diagnosis should be based
on wedge biopsy, the specimen may be taken from the
more peripheral, inflammatory part of the lesion alone.
In this case the diagnosis will be a false negative.
(Papanicolaou stain, x63).

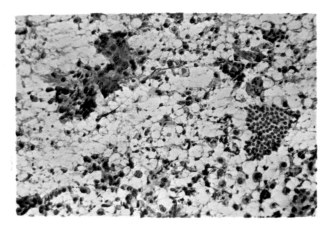

Fig. 12.5
In this case, the regular structure of the sheet of normal
ductal cells (right), contrasts markedly with the other
malignant cell population (isolated cells, necrotic background, clusters of atypical elements with loss of polarity).
(Papanicolaou stain, x63).

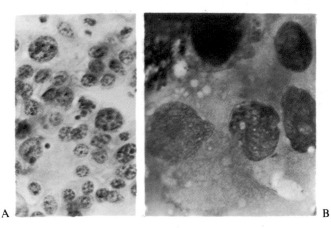

A   B

Fig. 12.6
Fine-needle aspirates from *poorly-differentiated adeno-*
carcinomas of the pancreas (in A, the aspiration was
performed at laparotomy, in B, percutaneously, with
ultrasonic guidance).
In A and B, the malignant cells form clusters which are
variable in thickness; these cells are highly pleomorphic,
with unevenly thickened nuclear membranes, coarse
chromocenters and prominent nucleoli.
(A: Papanicolaou stain, x250; B: M.G.G. stain, x600).

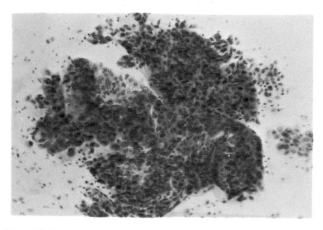

Fig. 12.7
This preparation was made with some fluid aspirated,
with a fine-needle, from a polycystic pancreatic mass
(filter imprint technique). Note pseudo-papillary fragments formed by multilayered malignant, fairly well-preserved
cells. A diagnosis of pancreatic ***papillary cystadenocarci-
noma*** was made.
(Papanicolaou stain, x250).

13
SPLEEN

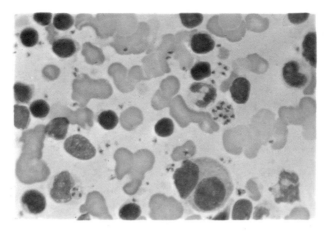

Fig. 13.1
Fine-needle spleen aspirate taken from a subject with *visceral leishmaniasis:* note intracellular and extracellular parasites *Leishmanias (donovani)*, which, at this magnification, are easily recognized; they are round-shaped and show a deeply red-stained corpuscle, corresponding to the nucleus. The kinetoplasts are only visible at a magnification greater than x1000.
(M.G.G. stain, x600).

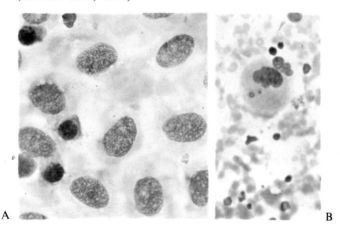

A   B

Fig. 13.2
Fine-needle aspirate in a subject with *myelosclerosis* and *splenic myeloid metaplasia.*
In A, the splenic fine-needle aspirate contains an inadvertently collected sheet of peritoneal cells; note normal mesothelial cells and three late normoblasts.
In B: lymphoid cells, immature cells of the neutrophil leucocyte series and one megakaryocyte.
(A: M.G.G. stain, x630; B: M.G.G. stain, x250).

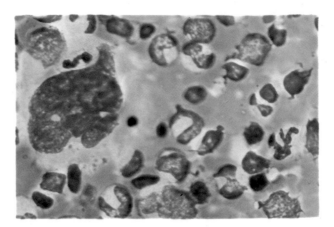

Fig. 13.3
A case of *splenic myeloid metaplasia*: one megakaryocyte, some normoblasts and more numerous immature cells of the neutrophil leucocyte series.
(M.G.G. stain, x600).

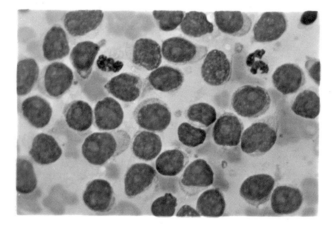

Fig. 13.4
Splenic fine-needle aspirate: monomorphic malignant lymphoid cells showing macronucleoli. In the blood-smears, a high percentage of similar cells were noted. The splenic cytologic picture was believed to indicate *prolymphocytic leukemia*.
(M.G.G. stain, x600).

14
KIDNEY

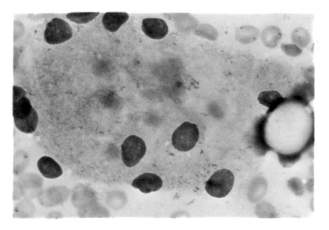

Fig. 14.1
Fine-needle aspirate from *normal renal parenchyma*. The
sheet probably corresponds to a proximal convoluted
tubule; round nuclei are surrounded by abundant cytoplasm, where fine, pink granules are present.
(M.G.G. stain, x600).

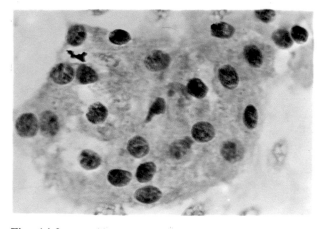

Fig. 14.2
Fine-needle aspirate from *normal renal parenchyma;* note
a sheet of cohesive cells, probably corresponding to a
proximal convoluted tubule. Note round and ovoid nuclei
with coarse but evenly distributed chromocenters; the
cytoplasm is abundant with indistinct boundaries and
pink granules.
(Papanicolaou stain, x600).

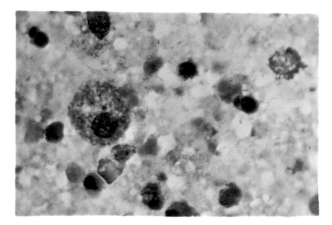

Fig. 14.3
Fine-needle aspirate (performed under ultrasonic guidance) from a renal mass, diagnosed as **solitary cyst**. Note necrotic debris (? neutrophils) and one histiocyte.
(M.G.G. stain, x600).

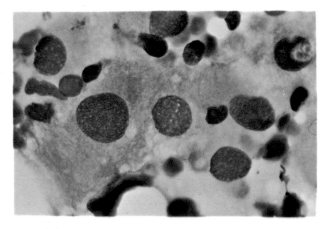

Fig. 14.4
Fine-needle aspirate from a renal mass, performed under ultrasonic guidance.
Note epithelial, malignant cells, characterized by fairly monomorphic nuclei, surrounded by abundant, sometimes foamy cytoplasm with indistinct boundaries and unevenly distributed granules. A diagnosis of **hypernephroma** was made (histologically confirmed).
(M.G.G. stain, x600).

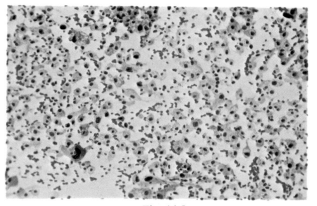

Fig. 14.5

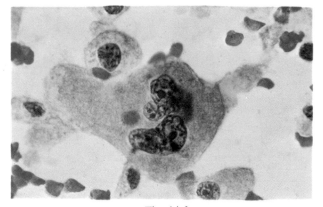

Fig. 14.6

Figs. 14.5 and 14.6
Fine-needle aspirate from a renal mass (*hypernephroma*),
performed at surgery. Note (Fig. 14.5) numerous malignant cells exhibiting moderate variability in shape and
size; they are mostly isolated and characterized by small
(sometimes multiple) hyperchromatic nuclei and granular
cytoplasm.
In Figure 14.6, at a higher magnification, the characteristic granular cytoplasm of some neoplastic cells can be
observed. These may be intermingled with, or completely
substitute, the more usual, clear cells. (The "clear"
appearance of the hypernephroma cells is due to the
scarcity of cytoplasmic organelles and to eluition of lipid
and glycogen during histologic processing; the "granular"
appearance is due to a peculiar richness of mitochondria
and cytosomes and to a more highly-developed endopla-
smic reticulum).
(Fig. 14.5: Papanicolaou stain, x63; Fig. 14.6: Papanicolaou stain, x630).

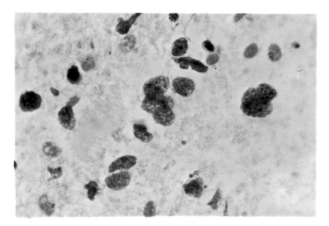

Fig. 14.7
Fine-needle aspirate from a renal mass, performed under
ultrasonic guidance. Note the poorly-differentiated malignant cells reduced to irregular, naked nuclei, sometimes
isolated, but mostly crowded and tightly packed. The
background is necrotic. This picture may correspond to
the more undifferentiated component of a *Wilms' tumor*
(the cytologic diagnosis was histologically confirmed).
(Papanicolaou stain, x600).

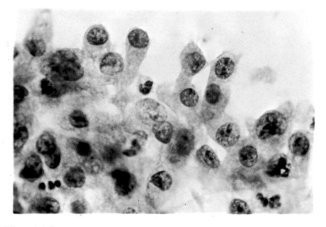

Fig. 14.8
Fine-needle aspirate from a mass in the renal pelvis,
performed under ultrasonic guidance. Numerous malignant, moderately differentiated cells, are depicted. Note
the cytoplasmic elongations characteristic of urothelial
tumors. A diagnosis of *transitional cell carcinoma* was
made (histologically confirmed).
(Papanicolaou stain, x600).

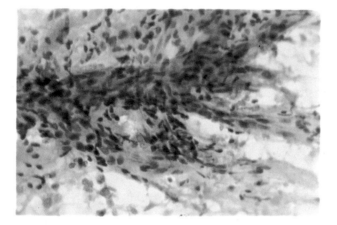

Fig. 14.9
Fine-needle aspirate from a renal mass, performed under ultrasonic guidance. Note bundles of spindle cells, moderately pleomorphic, intermingled with fat cells and droplets of fat.
A diagnosis of *renal angiomyolipoma* was made. Distinction should be made between this type of lesion and fibrosarcomatoid renal adenocarcinoma.
(Papanicolaou stain, x125).

15
RETROPERITONEUM

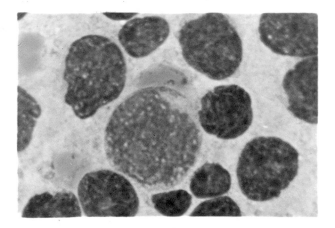

Fig. 15.1
Fine-needle aspirate from a retroperitoneal mass, performed under ultrasonic guidance: malignant tissue, formed
of variable-sized lymphoid cells, which sometimes show
cleaved nuclei.
A diagnosis of *malignant lymphoma, n.o.s.,* was made.
(M.G.G. stain, x1250).

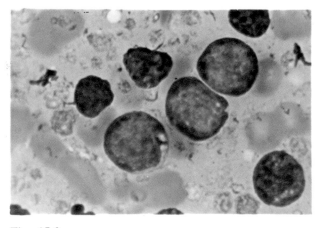

Fig. 15.2
Fine-needle aspirate from a retroperitoneal mass, performed under ultrasonic guidance. The case is similar to
that depicted in Figure 15.1 but the cells are more
monomorphic with very scanty cytoplasm and show some
nuclear vacuoles. A cytologic diagnosis of *(? lymphoblastic) lymphoma* was made.
(M.G.G. stain, x1250).

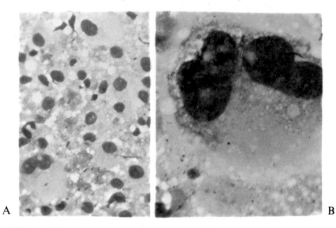

A   B

Fig. 15.3
Fine-needle aspirate from a retroperitoneal mass, performed under ultrasonic guidance. Note clusters of malignant
cells, which suggest an epithelial origin. In A and B,
multinucleated cells with clear, vacuolated, abundant
cytoplasm are also present.
A diagnosis of probable carcinoma metastasis was made
(the primary tumor was later identified as a *transitional
cell carcinoma*).
(A: M.G.G. stain, x125; B: M.G.G. stain, x600).

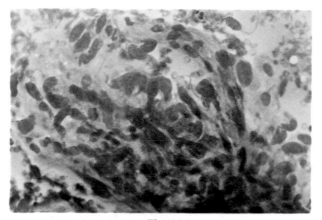

Fig. 15.4

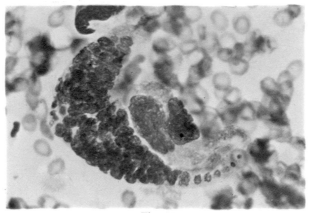

Fig. 15.5

Figs. 15.4 and 15.5
Fine-needle aspirate from a retroperitoneal mass, performed under ultrasonic guidance.
Note in Figure 15.4, malignant, parallel, spindle-cells,
arranged in bundles; the picture suggests a sarcomatous
lesion. In Figure 15.5, two malignant giant-cells, one of
which is ovoid and binucleated and the other crescent-
shaped, show innumerable, small, superposed nuclei. A
diagnosis of malignant mesenchymal tumor (possibly
primary) of the retroperitoneum (probably *malignant
fibrous histiocytoma*) was made and histologically confirmed).
(Fig. 15.4: M.G.G. stain, x250; Fig. 15.5: M.G.G. stain,
x600).

16
TESTIS

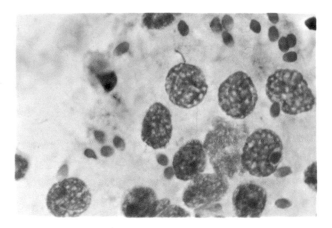

Fig. 16.1
Fine-needle aspirate from a *normal, sexually-mature testis*: note spermatozoa and spermatogonia. The latter show round nuclei, prominent nucleoli and indistinct cytoplasm.
(M.G.G. stain, x630).

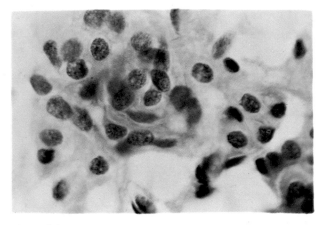

Fig. 16.2
Fine-needle aspirate from a palpable lesion of the testis, diagnosed as a non-specific, chronic, inflammatory disease.
Note a sheet of cohesive, ovoid or somewhat elongated cells; the nuclear structure is characterized by little, symmetrically arranged chromocenters; when present, the nucleoli are prominent. These cells were thought to be Sertoli cells; the high incidence of this type of cell suggests *chronic, inflammatory disease, with atrophy of the spermatogenic cells.*
(Papanicolaou stain, x600).

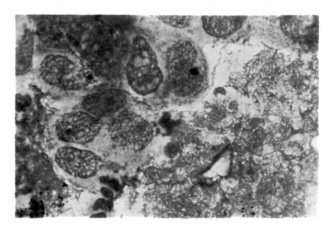

Fig. 16.3
Fine-needle aspirate from a painful, palpable lesion of
the testis: note necrotic debris, some neutrophils and a
cohesive sheet formed by Sertoli cells. A diagnosis of
acute, suppurative orchitis was made. Favourable outcome.
(M.G.G. stain, x630).

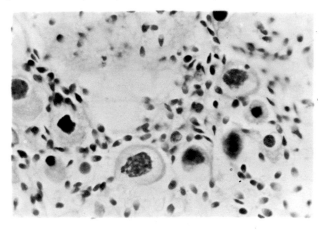

Fig. 16.4
This preparation was made with some fluid (approximately 10 ml) obtained by fine-needle aspiration from a
palpable testicular lesion, which turned out to be a cyst.
Note innumerable spermatozoa, intermingled with spermatogonia and histiocytes, with irregularly shaped and
hyperchromatic nuclei (these features are regressive and
not indicative of malignancy).
A cytologic diagnosis of ***spermatocele*** was made.
(Cytocentrifuge, Papanicolaou stain, x600).

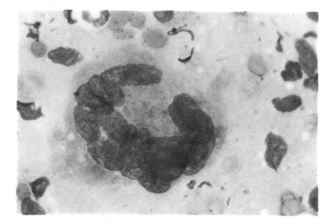

Fig. 16.5
Fine-needle aspirate from a palpable testicular lesion,
which was suspected to be malignant, on clinical grounds.
Smears made with cellular material obtained from various
points in the lesion always indicated chronic, inflammatory disease of the granulomatous type. Note inflammatory
cells and a giant, multinucleated histiocyte.
A cytologic diagnosis of **_granulomatous orchitis_** was made
(histologically confirmed).
(M.G.G. stain, x600).

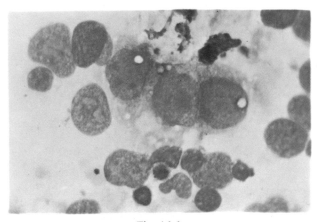

Fig. 16.6

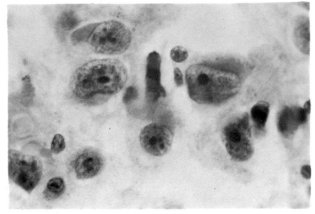

Fig. 16.7

Figs. 16.6 and 16.7
Two cases of *anaplastic-type seminomas*. The malignant
cells are polymorphous, dyshesive, the nuclei round or
ovoid, the nucleoli prominent. The cytoplasm is sometimes lacking because of the peculiar fragility of tumor
cells; the lymphocytes are sparse.
(Fig. 16.6: M.G.G. stain, x600; Fig. 16.7: Papanicolaou
stain, x600).

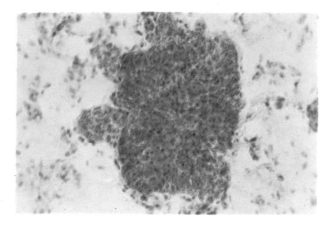

Fig. 16.8
Fine-needle aspirate from an *embryonal carcinoma* of the testis. These neoplasms are characterized by the abundant material usually collected at aspiration. The malignant cells are arranged in cohesive clusters, unlike seminoma cells which usually appear dyshesive.
In the case depicted above, a malignant, three-dimensional cluster and necrotic background can be noted. The cytologic details are more evident in Figures 16.9 and 16.10.
(Papanicolaou stain, x125).

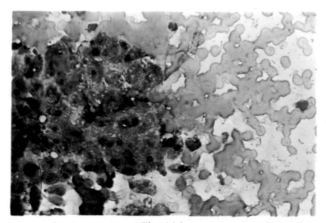

Fig. 16.9

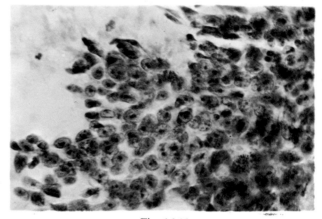

Fig. 16.10

Figs. 16.9 and 16.10
Fine-needle aspirate from an *embryonal carcinoma* of the
testis: note cohesive, three-dimensional clusters, formed
by predominantly ovoid, monomorphic cells, with large
nuclei, a thickened nuclear membrane and prominent
nucleoli. The cytoplasm appears better-preserved than in
seminomas.
(Fig. 16.9: M.G.G. stain, x250; Fig. 16.10: Papanicolaou
stain, x250).

17
PROSTATE

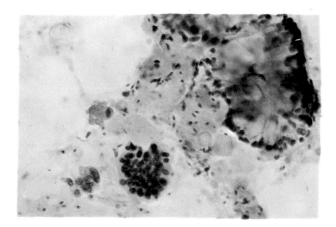

Fig. 17.1
Contaminants collected during prostatic fine-needle aspiration: rectal mucosa (tall columnar cells, with peripherically situated nuclei), cells of seminal vesicles, sperm and
talc.
(Papanicolaou stain, x125).

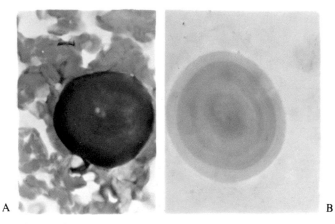

A   B

Fig. 17.2
A: Rounded, laminated structure observed in a fine-needle
prostatic aspirate: it corresponds to an ***amylaceous body***,
blue stained with M.G.G.
B: An ***amylaceous body*** in Papanicolaou preparation; it
shows a concentrically laminated structure.
(A: M.G.G. stain, x600; B: Papanicolaou stain, x600).

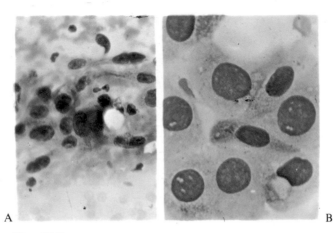

A   B

Fig. 17.3
The cells depicted in A and B show the features most
frequently observed in *elements from seminal vesicles;*
they are columnar or ovoid-columnar and the cytoplasm
contains pink granules.
(A: M.G.G. stain, x250; B: M.G.G. stain, x600).

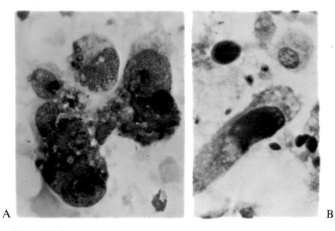

A   B

Fig. 17.4
The cells depicted in A and B are *benign elements from
seminal vesicles;* the nuclei are huge and hyperchromatic.
Very characteristic the cytoplasmic yellow-brown pig-
ment.
(A: M.G.G. stain, x600; B: Papanicolaou stain, x600).

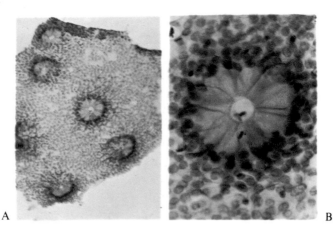

A   B

Fig. 17.5
In A and B, *acinar sheet (from normal prostate);* the
hollow spaces correspond to proximal ductal structures.
The prostatic cells, depicted in B, are observed laterally
and from above. This feature may lead to their erroneous
interpretation as elements from the rectal mucosa
(contaminants).
(A: Papanicolaou stain, x63; B: Papanicolaou stain, x250).

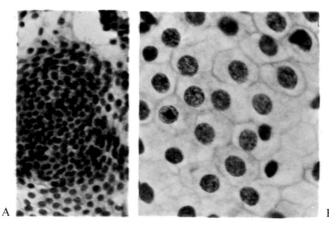

A   B

Fig. 17.6
In A, a sheet of prostatic cells with a vorticose appearance
where the cells overlap, because of being forcibly ejected
onto the slide. These features must be well-known to
avoid false positives.
Note, in B, a monolayered honeycombed sheet of normal
prostatic cells; they are polyhedral and the cytoplasmic
edges are sharp. This epithelial sheet is derived from a
hyperplastic nodule, but it is undistinguishable from
"normal" prostatic epithelium. The diagnosis of hyperplastic disease should be made on the base of clinical
evidence.
(A: Papanicolaou stain, x125; B: Papanicolaou stain,
x600).

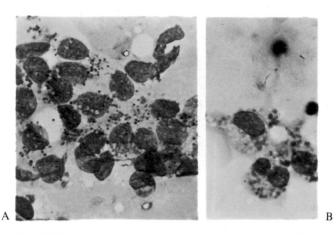

A   B

Fig. 17.7
Fine-needle aspirate from a *prostatic nodule due to benign hyperplasia*.
Note, in A, uneven, flattened, glandular cells on which red secretive granules are superposed: in B, three phagocytizing histiocytes with foamy cytoplasm.
(A, B: M.G.G. stain, x600).

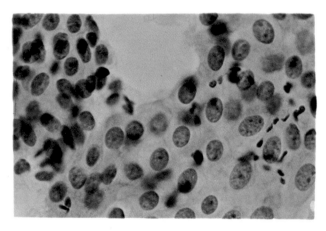

Fig. 17.8
Group of *hyperplastic multilayered glandular cells* with mostly evident nucleoli. Neutrophils are also present (more numerous elsewhere in the slide). Such a picture suggests acute prostatitis, and the epithelial cells are probably of the repair type.
(Papanicolaou stain, x250).

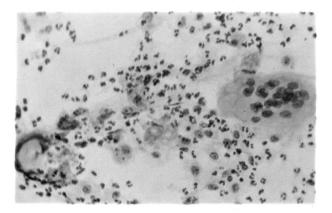

Fig. 17.9
Fine-needle aspirate from an irregular, firm prostatic
nodule, highly suspected of malignancy, on clinical
grounds: the lesion is granulomatous in type: note the
giant multinucleated cell, histiocytes and innumerable
neutrophils. A diagnosis of ***granulomatous prostatitis*** was
made. Unremarkable follow-up for two years.
(Papanicolaou stain, x250).

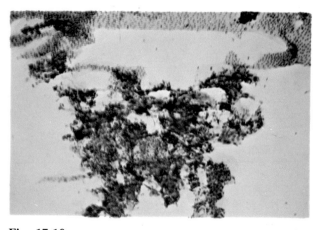

Fig. 17.10
Fine-needle aspirate from ***prostatic adenocarcinoma;*** at
low magnification, the benign, ribbon-like, monolayered,
horizontally placed sheet (top) can easily be distinguished
from the malignant, disorderly arranged, multilayered
cells (bottom).
(Papanicolaou stain, x20).

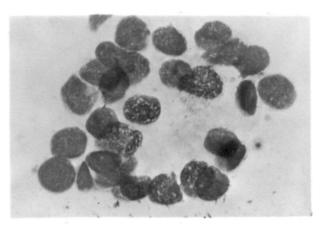

Fig. 17.11
Well-differentiated, prostatic adenocarcinoma: note characteristic microacinar structure. The cytoplasm is crowded in a central mass, and the nuclei arranged in a peripheral circle. Anisonucleosis is not marked, the nucleoli are rare.
In well-differentiated, prostatic adenocarcinoma, the diagnosis is suggested by a cytologic pattern characterised by (almost) exclusive microacini, instead of the glandular sheets, which are observed in benign prostatic enlargements.
(M.G.G. stain, x600).

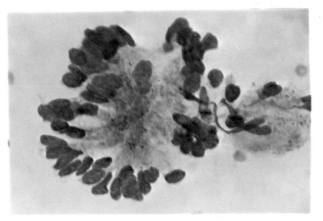

Fig. 17.12
Fine-needle aspirate from prostatic tumor, diagnosed as *endometrioid carcinoma of the utriculus mascularus.* Note a microacinar-papillary structure formed by tall, columnar, monomorphic cells, with small, peripheral nuclei. The neoplasm was deeply-infiltrating of the surrounding glandular parenchyma.
(M.G.G. stain, x250).

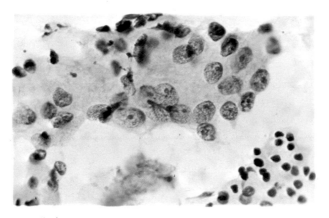

Fig. 17.13
Fine-needle aspirate from a symmetrically enlarged prostate, which physical examination suggested to be hyperplastic. Note a cohesive epithelial sheet with partially overlapping nuclei and loss of polarity; there is slight anisonucleosis, the nuclear membranes are thickened and eosinophilic nucleoli are prominent.
For comparison, observe the features of a glandular benign sheet (lower-right corner).
A diagnosis of ***moderately-differentiated, prostatic adenocarcinoma*** was made (histologically confirmed).
(Papanicolaou stain, x630).

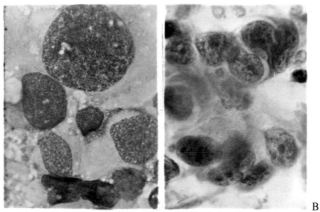

A   B

Fig. 17.14
Fine-needle aspirate from a ***poorly-differentiated, adenocarcinoma.*** In A and B, there are no glandular structures. Especially in B, marked poikilocytosis; the malignant cells are multilayered, the nuclear-cytoplasmic ratio is increased, the nuclear membranes are irregularly thickened, the chromocenters hyperchromatic and the nucleoli prominent.
(A: M.G.G. stain, x600; B: Papanicolaou stain, x600).

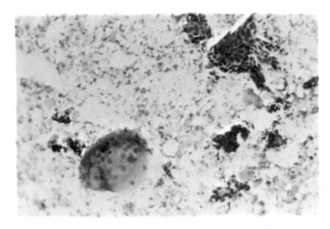

Fig. 17.15
Fine-needle aspirate from a complex, prostatic lesion:
note a giant, multinucleated cell, the necrotic and
inflammatory background, and (on the right) the numerous epithelial groups, characterized by multilayering and
loss of polarity in peripheral nuclei. A diagnosis of
**granulomatous prostatitis associated with moderately-
differentiated adenocarcinoma** was made.
(Papanicolaou stain, x125).

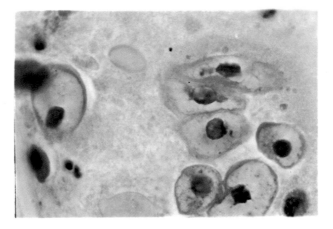

Fig. 17.16
Fine-needle aspirate of the prostate in a patient affected
by **(estrogen-treated) adenocarcinoma**.
The response to hormone therapy was judged good,
because of the fairly-exclusive presence of squamous
metaplastic (non-malignant) cells (no cancer cells present
elsewhere in the slides.)
(Papanicolaou stain, x600).

18
OVARY

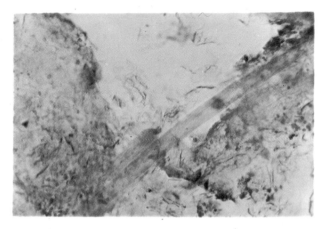

Fig. 18.1
Fine-needle aspirate from a large ovarian cyst, obtained transvaginally. Note the heterogeneous picture, characterised by amorphous debris, hair, non-nucleated squamae. A diagnosis of *ovarian teratoma (dermoid cyst)* was made. (Papanicolaou stain, x125).

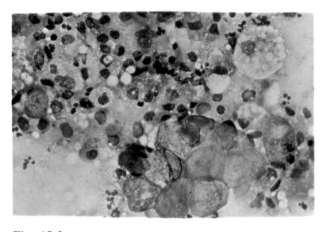

Fig. 18.2
Fine-needle aspirate from an ovarian cyst, diagnosed as *dermoid cyst*: numerous inflammatory cells (neutrophils, lymphocytes, histiocytes) and a group of non-nucleated squamae.
(Papanicolaou stain, x250).

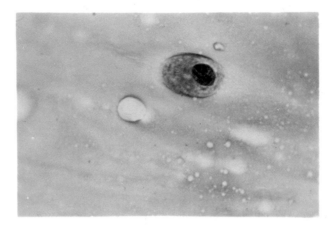

Fig. 18.3
Fine-needle aspirate from an ovarian mass, diagnosed as
mucinous cystoma: note bluish substance in the background (mucus) and an epithelial, columnar cell, with a
basal, fairly well-preserved nucleus.
(M.G.G. stain, x600).

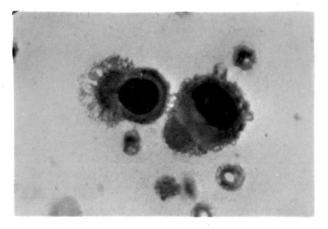

Fig. 18.4
Fine-needle aspirate from an ovarian "cystic" lesion,
obtained under ultrasonic guidance (a small quantity of
fluid containing a few cells was withdrawn). The cells are
roundish, fairly monomorphic with ciliated, pseudopodia-
like, cytoplasmic protrusions; these elements are not
clearly malignant. A cytological diagnosis of *ovarian
cystoadenoma* was made.
(Cytocentrifuge, M.G.G. stain, x600).

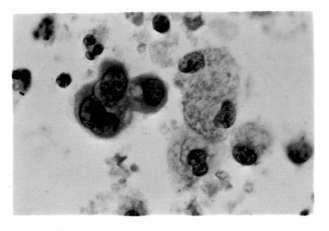

Fig. 18.5
Fine-needle aspirate from an ovarian cyst, obtained under
ultrasonic guidance. Note the small cluster of roundish
and columnar-shaped, epithelial cells, exhibiting thick
nuclear membranes and prominent nucleoli, intermingled
with macrophages and neutrophils. A cytologic diagnosis
of a ***possible serous cystoadenoma with inflammatory
changes*** was made.
(Papanicolaou stain, x600).

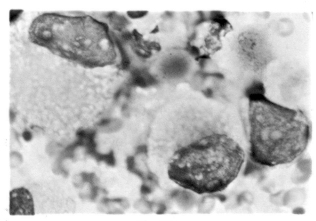

Fig. 18.6

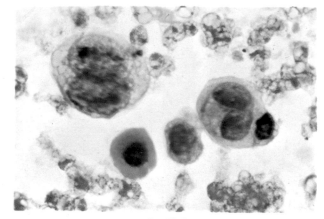

Fig. 18.7

Figs. 18.6 and 18.7
In Figure 18.6, fine-needle aspirate from an ovarian polycystic mass: the epithelial cells are fairly numerous and larger than those of Figure 18.3. The nuclei are peripherally situated and the cytoplasm contains microvacuoles. In the midfield, note the presence of structureless blue-stained material (mucus). A diagnosis of **mucinous cystoadenocarcinoma** was made (histologically confirmed).
In Figure 18.7, other cells from the previous case are depicted; they exhibit marked variability in size, irregular nuclei (pyknosis, multiple nuclei) and cytoplasmic vacuoles.
(Fig. 18.6: M.G.G. stain, x600; Fig. 18.7: Papanicolaou stain, x600).

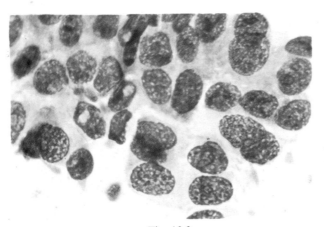

Fig. 18.8

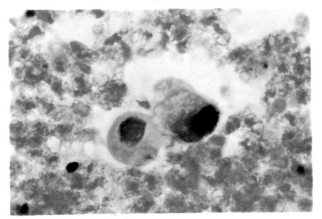

Fig. 18.9

Figs. 18.8 and 18.9
Fine-needle aspirate from an ovarian mass, diagnosed as
serous cystoadenocarcinoma. Note in Figure 18.8, polymorphous, epithelial cells arranged to form a papillary-
like structure; they appear smaller than those of mucinous
cystoadenocarcinoma, as depicted in Figure 18.6. Elsewhere in the slide, some psammoma bodies are present.
In Figure 18.9, the same case as Figure 18.8: note two
malignant cells, exhibiting marked regressive aspects.
(Fig. 18.8: M.G.G. stain, x600; Fig. 18.9: Papanicolaou
stain, x600).

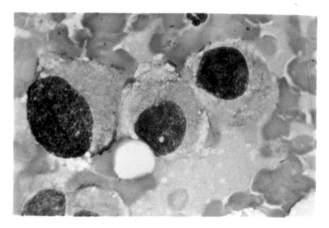

Fig. 18.10
Fine-needle aspirate from an ovarian mass, obtained under ultrasonic guidance; note a high concentration of malignant cells, which are fairly monomorphic; the nuclear atypias are more marked than those of the cells depicted in Figure 18.6. A diagnosis of ***poorly-differentiated ovarian carcinoma*** was made.
(M.G.G. stain, x630).

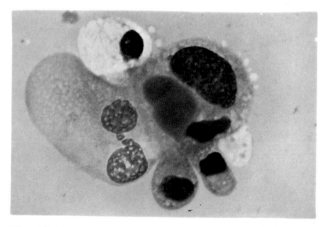

Fig. 18.11
Fine-needle aspirate from an ovarian mass, performed under ultrasonic guidance: note malignant epithelial cells, characterized by large cytoplasm with small vacuoles and marked anisonucleosis. They are arranged in an acinar-like structure, in which a deeply-red stained drop of mucus is evident.
A diagnosis of ***clear-cell (mesonephroid) adenocarcinoma*** was made.
(M.G.G. stain, x600).

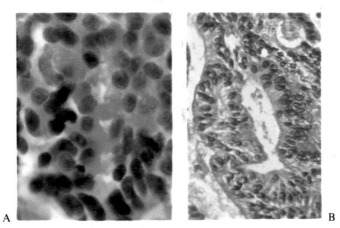

A   B

Fig. 18.12
Fine-needle aspirate from an ovarian mass, obtained
under ultrasonic guidance: note, in A, a three-dimensional, malignant cluster formed by epithelial, hyperchromatic, rather monomorphic cells; in B, histologic section
obtained by paraffin embedding of small fragments
aspirated with fine-needle; with the use of the latter
technique, the endometrial-like architecture of the neoplasm is more evident than in the cytological picture
exhibited in A.
A diagnosis of *endometrioid adenocarcinoma of the ovary*
was made (histologically confirmed).
(A, B: Papanicolaou stain, x250).

19

SOFT PARTS AND MISCELLANEOUS LESIONS

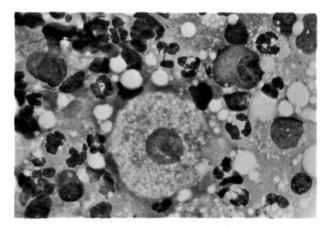

Fig. 19.1
Fine-needle aspirate from a palpable gluteal mass. Note variable-sized histiocytes, innumerable neutrophils, lymphocytes, plasmacells and hollow structures (corresponding to fatty tissue). This cytologic picture suggests a *chronic inflammatory process of the subcutaneous tissue.* Favourable outcome.
(M.G.G. stain, x600).

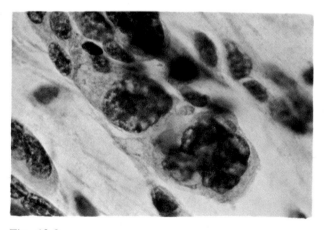

Fig. 19.2
Fine-needle aspirate from a mass in the forearm soft tissues: the obviously malignant cytologic picture is characterized by the presence of predominantly spindle-shaped, parallel cells arranged in bundles; in the midfield, note two polyploid malignant cells. In this case, the only possible cytologic diagnosis is *probable sarcomatous lesion (n.o.s.).* The final diagnosis must be based on histologic findings.
(Papanicolaou stain, x600).

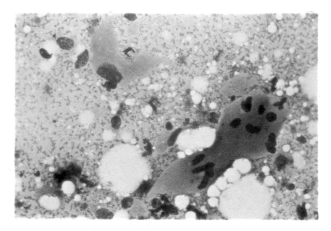

Fig. 19.3
Fine-needle aspirate from a sternocleidomastoid lump,
which developed after radiation therapy for cervical
metastasis from carcinoma. Background of inflammatory
cells and two atrophic muscle fibers, showing apparent
sarcolemmal polynucleosis. A cytologic diagnosis of
actinic myositis was made.
(M.G.G. stain, x250).

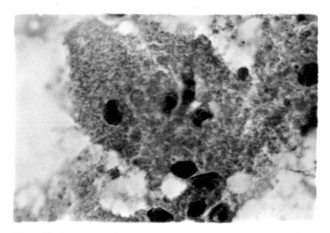

Fig. 19.4
Fine-needle aspirate from a breast lump, suspected of
malignancy, on clinical grounds; the cells are monomorphic with indistinct boundaries, small, hyperchromatic,
peripherically situated nuclei and diffusely granular
cytoplasm. A diagnosis of *granular cell myoblastoma* was
made (histologically confirmed).
(Papanicolaou stain, x600).

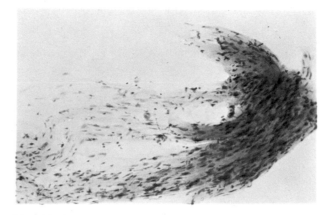

Fig. 19.5
Fine-needle aspirate from supraclavicular lump: aspiration was painful (giving an "electric shock" sensation, in the homolateral arm). Note a sheet of cohesive spindle-shaped cells (with round nuclear ends) arranged in parallel bundles. A cytological diagnosis of *schwannoma* was made (histologically confirmed on tissue-section of a neoplasm removed from the brachial plexus).
(Papanicolaou stain, x63).

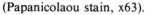

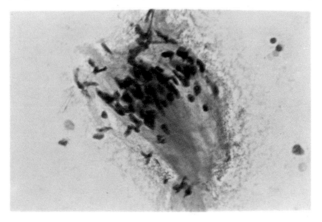

Fig. 19.6
Fine-needle aspirate from a *schwannoma*: "fibrillar" fragment showing small nuclei arranged in palisades. Such a structure could correspond to a Verocay body.
(Papanicolaou stain, x250).

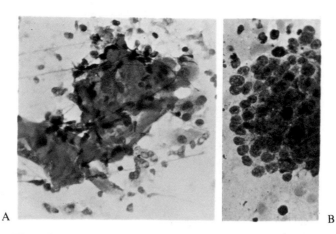

A   B

Fig. 19.7
Fine-needle aspirate from a nodular skin lesion; in A, small, monomorphic, cohesive or isolated, epithelial cells (basal cells), intermingled with eosinophilic, structureless material (squamous, ghost-cells).
In B, basal cohesive cells, exhibiting prominent nucleoli.
A diagnosis of *calcifying epithelioma of Malherbe (pilomatrixoma)* was made (histologically confirmed).
(A: Papanicolaou stain, x125; B: M.G.G. stain, x125).

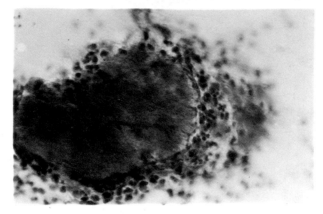

Fig. 19.8
Fine-needle aspirate from a suprahyoid mass, clinically diagnosed as acute inflammatory lesion: "sulphur granule" enveloped by innumerable, partly-lysed neutrophils *(actinomycosis)*. The mycelia are orangeophilic.
(Papanicolaou stain, x400).

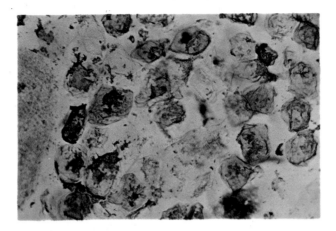

Fig. 19.9
Fine-needle aspirate from a cervical mass: 1 ml of viscid
yellow fluid was withdrawn. Note the exclusive presence
of disintegrating sebaceous cells. A diagnosis of *sebaceous
cyst* was made.
(M.G.G. stain, x250).

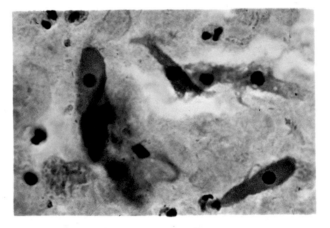

Fig. 19.10
Fine-needle aspirate from a cervical mass: epidermoid,
eosinophilic nucleated cells, neutrophils, granular debris.
A diagnosis of *epidermal inclusion cyst (with acute,
superimposed inflammation)* was made. In congenital,
lateral cysts of the neck, the epidermoidal cells may
sometimes show marked atypias, and the differential
diagnosis between congenital cyst and (liquefied) metastasis of a well-differentiated epidermoid carcinoma may be
difficult.
(Papanicolaou stain, x600).

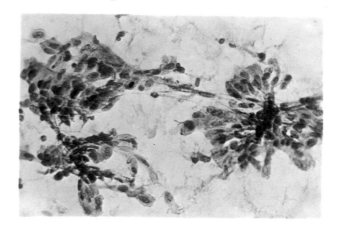

Fig. 19.11
Fine-needle aspirate from a suprahyoid mass: 2 ml of
yellow fluid were withdrawn. Note sheets of columnar
cells, sometimes showing cilia.
Medial congenital cysts of the neck may be lined with
squamous or columnar epithelium.
(Papanicolaou stain, x125).

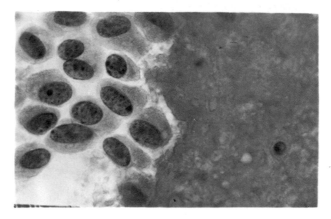

Fig. 19.12
Fine-needle aspirate from a post-traumatic abdominal
muscle mass. Note red blood cells and isolated, ovoid,
monomorphic cells, sometimes showing evident nucleoli;
the cytoplasm is large and acidophilic, with fairly sharp
edges. The latter cells are normal (i.e. not activated),
mesothelial cells, aspirated from parietal peritoneal lining.
A cytological diagnosis of *muscular hematoma* was made
(confirmed at surgery).
(Papanicolaou stain, x400).

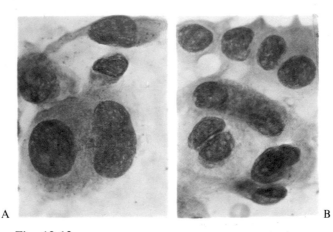

A   B

Fig. 19.13
Fine-needle aspirate from a subcutaneous, inguinal mass:
note malignant, sometimes binucleated cells which are
round, oval, spindle or polyhedral-shaped; the nuclei are
highly polymorphic; the cytoplasm shows occasional
microvacuoles and sometimes a filamentous appearance
(see spindle-shaped cell, in A).
Such a cytological picture corresponds to the **rhabdomyo-
sarcomatous component** of - a neoplasm which was
histologically classified as malignant mesenchymal mixed
tumor (so-called malignant mesenchymoma).
(A, B: M.G.G. stain, x630).

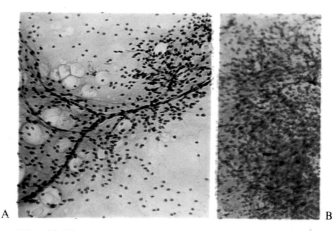

A   B

Fig. 19.14
Fine-needle aspirate from a popliteal mass (a popliteal
myxoid liposarcoma had previously been removed from
this region). The picture, characterized by a rich vascular
network of capillaries in a plexiform arrangement, is
similar to that of embryonal fat; the cells (not clearly
discernible, at this magnification) are mostly stellate. Such
a picture suggests a local recurrence of **myxoid liposarcoma**.
(A: Papanicolaou stain, x63; B: M.G.G. stain, x63).

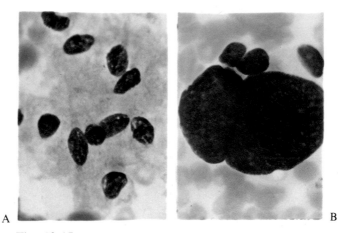

Fig. 19.15
Fine-needle aspirate from a cervical mass, clinically
diagnosed as lymphadenopathy: in A, the material
collected is represented by numerous blood red cells and
by cells with abundant cytoplasm and round or ovoid
nuclei; the cells are sometimes isolated, sometimes
arranged in little sheets; occasionally, follicular-like
structures can be seen; huge, hyperchromatic, naked
nuclei are also present (see B).
A diagnosis of *possible carotid body tumour (chemodecto-*
ma) was made (histologically confirmed). This type of
lesion must be distinguished from a possible metastasis
from a differentiated carcinoma of the thyroid.
(A: M.G.G. stain, x250; B: M.G.G. stain, x600).

20
BONE

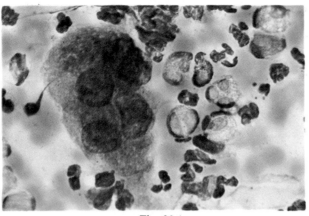

Fig. 20.1

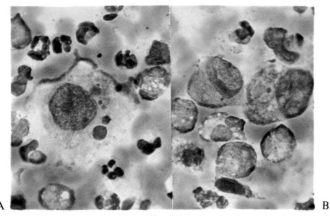

A   B

Fig. 20.2

Figs. 20.1 and 20.2
Fine-needle aspirate (performed under fluoroscopic guidance) from a lytic lesion of the mandible: note a granulomatous picture (neutrophils, eosinophils, mononucleated and multinucleated cells). In the latter (Langerhans' cells of histiocytosis-X), a deep, narrow folding of the nuclear membrane can be seen; in B of Figure 20.2, the phagocytized material in the right histiocyte consists, at least partly, of granules from eosinophils. A diagnosis of *eosinophilic granuloma of the bone* was made (histologically confirmed).
(Fig. 20.1: M.G.G. stain, x600; Fig. 20.2 A, B: M.G.G. stain, x600).

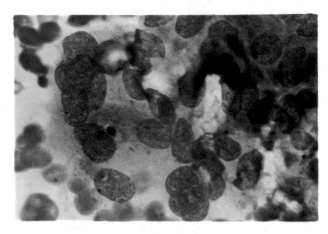

Fig. 20.3
Fine-needle aspirate from a lytic lesion of the mandible,
in a patient with parathyroid adenoma. This picture was
believed to correspond to the so-called *giant-cell repara-
tive granuloma (brown tumor):* note the giant multinucleated cell (osteoclast) next to other similar, superposed
elements.
(M.G.G. stain, x600).

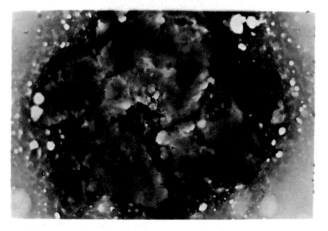

Fig. 20.4
Fine-needle aspirate from an *osteochondroma (osteocarti-
laginous exostosis):* note, in a bloody background, the
cloud-like mass of chondroid substance which varies in
color from pink to dark purple.
(M.G.G. stain, x125).

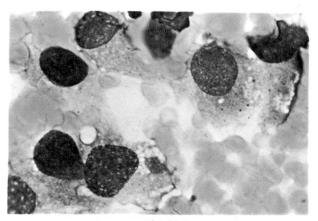

Fig. 20.5

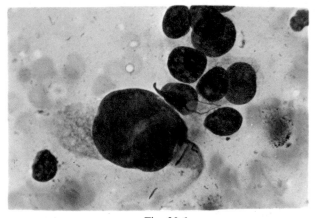

Fig. 20.6

Figs. 20.5 and 20.6

Fine-needle aspirate from an *osteosarcoma:* the malignant cells are mononucleated, the nuclei ovoid and eccentrically situated; there is mild anisonucleosis and the nuclear membranes are fairly evenly thickened. The chromocenters are fairly clumped, evenly distributed and the nucleoli (which are sometimes two per cell) evident. The cytoplasm is basophilic, with microvacuoles.

Note in Figure 20.6, a huge, polyploid, malignant cell. (Fig. 20.5: M.G.G. stain, x600; Fig. 20.6: M.G.G. stain, x600).

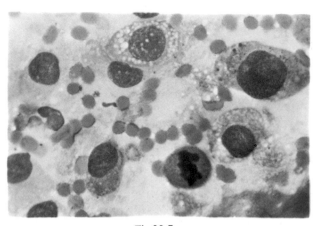

Fig.20.7

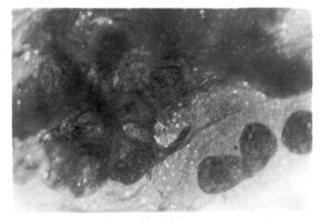

Fig. 20.8

Figs. 20.7 and 20.8
Cells aspirated from two *chondrosarcomas*. In Figure 20.7, in a bloody background, isolated, very atypical malignant cells are depicted. The nuclei are round or ovoid, fairly large, with coarse and irregular chromatin network. The nucleoli are sometimes multiple. The highly basophilic cytoplasm often contains microvacuoles. A malignant cell shows atypical mitosis. Note amorphous, reddish, chondroid material (lower-right corner).
In Figure 20.8, malignant cells with prominent nucleoli, next to a (myxo)chondroid substance are seen.
(Fig. 20.7: M.G.G. stain, x600; Fig. 20.8: M.G.G. stain, x600).

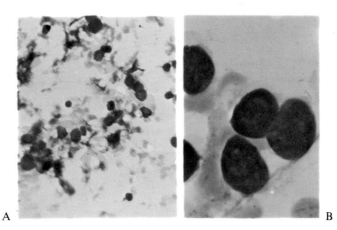

A   B

Fig. 20.9
Fine-needle aspirate from an *Ewing's sarcoma*. In A, the
malignant cells are isolated or cohesive; the (often naked)
nuclei are elliptic. In B, moderate anisonucleosis and
markedly clumped chromatin.
(A: M.G.G. stain, x125; B: M.G.G. stain, x600).

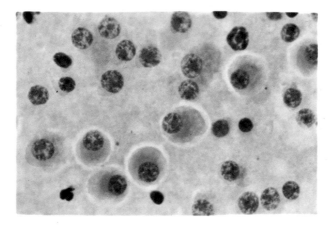

Fig. 20.10
Myeloma cells aspirated from a lytic lesion of the
skeleton; the malignant plasmacells show a granular,
chromatin network and, often, prominent nucleoli. There
is discrete anisocytosis. A diagnosis of *myeloma, moderately dedifferentiated type* was made.
(Papanicolaou stain, x600).

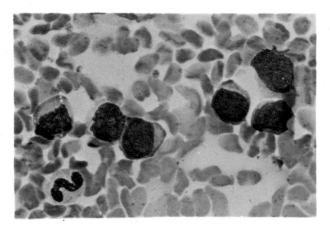

Fig. 20.11
Fine-needle aspirate from a lytic lesion of the mandible:
note isolated, monomorphic cells showing agranular
basophilic cytoplasm, large, roundish or cleaved nuclei
and prominent nucleoli. This picture was believed
compatible with *lymphomatous (n.o.s.) lesion of the bone*.
(M.G.G. stain, x600).

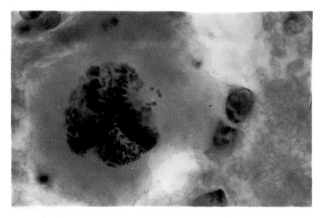

Fig. 20.12
Fine-needle aspirate from a lytic diaphyseal lesion of the
humerus (obtained under fluoroscopic guidance). There
are malignant cells with eosinophilic cytoplasm; among
them a giant, polyploid cell. A diagnosis of *bone
metastasis from epidermoid, well-differentiated carcinoma*
was made (elsewhere in the slide, horn pearls were
present).
(Papanicolaou stain, x630).

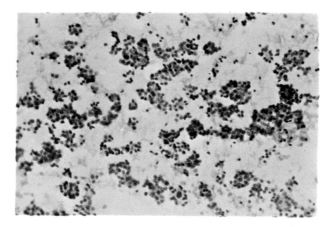

Fig. 20.13
Fine-needle aspirate from a lytic lesion of the pelvis. Note
malignant cells in microfollicular arrangement. In some
structures, an eosinophilic substance (colloid) is discernible. A diagnosis of ***bone metastasis from follicular thyroid
adenocarcinoma*** was made.
(Papanicolaou stain, x125).

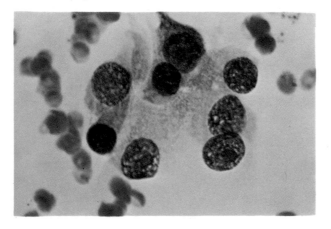

Fig. 20.14
Group of malignant cells aspirated from a lytic bone
lesion: the cells have roundish nuclei; the chromatin is
fairly coarse but evenly distributed; the nucleoli are
prominent; the cytoplasm is abundant and clear, with
distinct boundaries. A diagnosis of ***bone metastasis from
a clear-cell, renal adenocarcinoma*** was made.
(M.G.G. stain, x600).

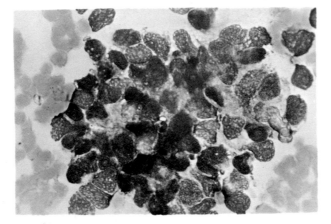

Fig. 20.15
Fine-needle aspirate from a lytic bone lesion. Note cluster
of small, malignant, epithelial cells, with irregular nuclei,
nucleoli and a small peripheral rim of cytoplasm. On the
left, a microacinar structure in clearly visible. A diagnosis
of ***bone metastasis possibly from a prostatic, well-
differentiated adenocarcinoma*** was made.
(M.G.G. stain, x600).